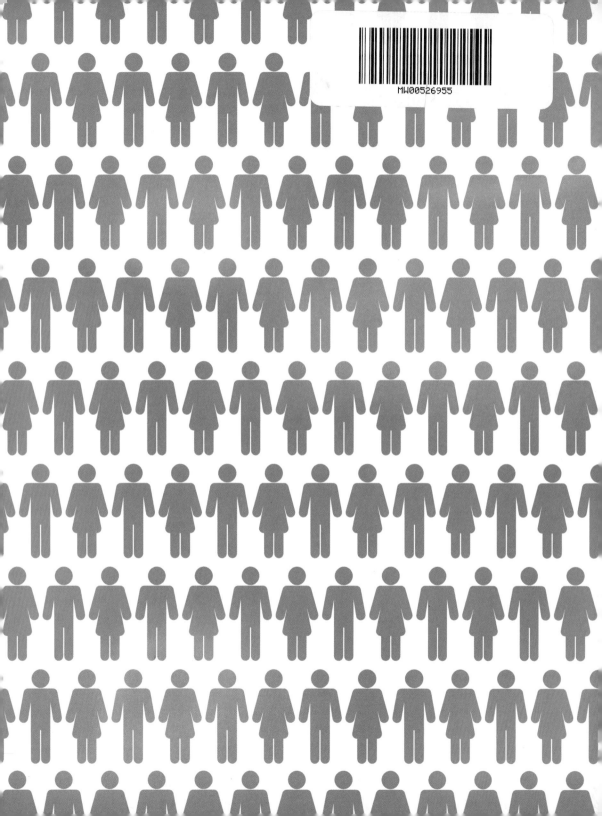

Love you! ♡

THE **T** GUIDE

Eren ♡
you are
Shung ♡ !
Yuji Yorgdaenko! ♡

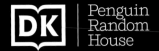

Penguin Random House

Publisher Mike Sanders
Art & Design Director William Thomas
Editor Brandon Buechley
Photographer Shaun Vadella
Illustrator Marco Marco

First American Edition, 2023
Published in the United States by DK Publishing
6081 E 82nd St., Indianapolis, IN 46250

The authorized representative in the EEA is Dorling Kindersley
Verlag GmbH. Arnulfstr. 124, 80636 Munich, Germany

A catalog record for this book
is available from the Library of Congress.
ISBN: 978-0-7440-7059-0

DK books are available at special discounts when purchased
in bulk for sales promotions, premiums, fund-raising, or educational use.
For details, contact: SpecialSales@dk.com.

Printed and bound in Italy.

For the curious
www.dk.com

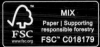

MIX
Paper | Supporting
responsible forestry
FSC™ C018179

This book was made with Forest
Stewardship Council ™ certified
paper - one small step in DK's
commitment to a sustainable future.
**For more information go to
www.dk.com/our-green-pledge**

THE T GUIDE

GIGI GORGEOUS & GOTTMIK

To all our trans siblings in the world. No matter where you are on your journey,

you are seen,
you are heard,
and you are loved.

We would also like to extend a special thank you
to Anthony Allen Ramos and GLAAD for their support.

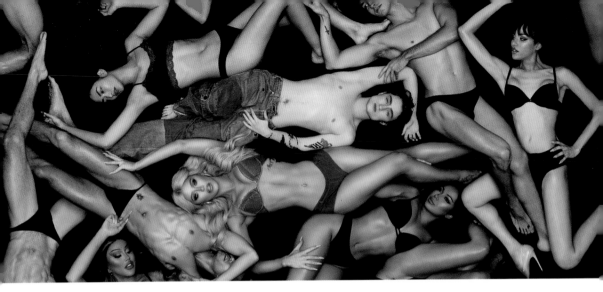

Contents

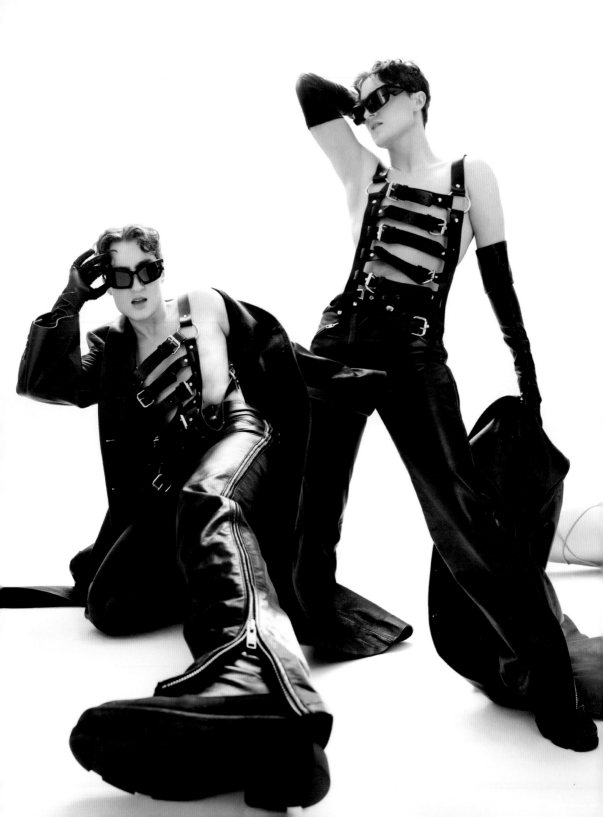

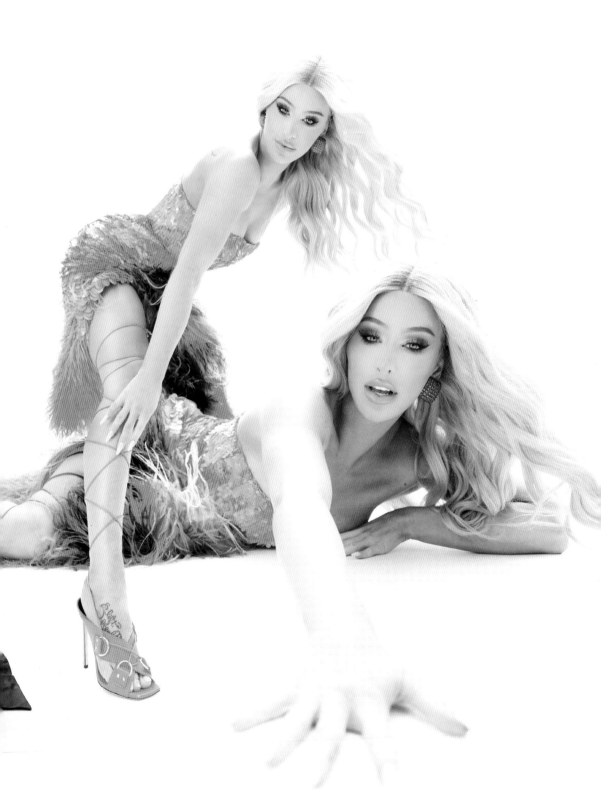

Introduction

Hey, Gorgeous!

Can you believe there isn't an awesome, informative guide to transitioning out there yet?

We couldn't either, so we decided to write one.

In this book, we're going to take you through the steps of the transitioning process—for people assigned F at birth and people assigned M at birth. (*F* and *M* stand for "female" and "male," in case you're new to this lingo!) Basically, this is all the information we wish we had when we were first starting out. We're going to tell you all the details about how we did it, and we've asked some friends to chime in as well so you can read about a bunch of different experiences. We've done our best to choose a really diverse group of people: old, young, famous, not, family members, allies … you get the point.

In these pages, we're going to try to be as informative as possible, and as loving. We are not here to gatekeep. We're going to divulge everything we know. Although many elements of the transitioning journey have been spectacularly developed, others have a ways to go. For example, facial feminization is a procedure you can get, but facial masculinization is not. Why? And how can you make up your own version of it? (Getting some jaw filler would be one step.)

What's special about this book is that it's written by two people who care about each other deeply, and who've helped each other through many moments of the transitioning process. We want to help you, too, and we want this book to be a tangible reminder that you can move forward, even if what's in front of you seems insurmountable. When you feel scared or discouraged, we want you to open this book and feel the love. We also want you to walk away with practical tips on how to transition, because this book is, after all, a guide—uniquely formatted as a conversation.

The trans experience has gotten more public attention recently, but we still have work to do. A lot of people in this country—and in the world—don't really understand what it actually means to be trans, or all that the concept of transitioning entails. So, if the people around you aren't getting you, that would make sense. Maybe after you read this book, you can buy them a copy. This book is for allies, parents, and anyone who is looking to educate themselves on the trans experience.

There are so many choices to make when you're transitioning, and everyone's journey is unique. We hope that this book inspires you to carve out your own confident path. At the very least, we want you to feel some ease after reading this.

You are not alone.

Because we, Gigi and Gottmik, are your new best friends.

Gigi Gorgeous ♡.   *Gottmik*

A Disclaimer

We are not experts. We're sharing our opinions based on our personal experience. Ultimately, you are the one who knows what's best for you. Please take only what you find useful from this book and leave the rest.

Gigi Gorgeous *on*
Gottmik

Gottmik is one of the funniest, most original, sensitive, thoughtful, wildly creative people I know. I met him out of drag, as Kade, at a club around 2016. One of our friends was like, "Oh my God, you should do Gigi's makeup!" We just clicked instantly. Then Kade and my husband, Nats, became super close. They both transitioned around the same time, which bonded them in a special way.

When Gottmik was given the opportunity to be the first trans male contestant on *RuPaul's Drag Race,* he seriously rose to the occasion. I was so impressed! He was knowledgeable and graceful, and he spoke so eloquently about the community. Not only is Gottmik a lovable and compelling TV star, he's also an insanely talented makeup artist. He was a star behind the camera, and now he's a star in front of the camera. I knew from the moment I met him that he was destined for all this success.

Gottmik *on*
Gigi Gorgeous

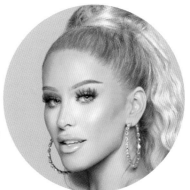

The first time I saw Gigi on YouTube, I was awestruck. I couldn't believe that someone was sharing about their transition in such an open, honest way. Gigi was groundbreaking on that platform. Nobody else was doing what she was doing. Then she made her documentary, *This Is Everything: Gigi Gorgeous,* and the trailer went viral, and there were billboards with her face on them all over LA. By making her personal story public, she really humanized the transitioning process to a mass audience, which was a huge gift to the community. Her bravery has been inspiring to a lot of people, me included.

Getting to know Gigi has been such a privilege. The thing I admire most about her is that she lives with such ease. Even when she's doing things that are hard, she makes them seem like no big deal. Her positive outlook is magnetic. She's always in the mood to have fun, and she's such a supportive friend.

I met Gigi right at the time when I was starting to seriously question my identity. At first, I wasn't sure how much I wanted to share about it, and she was like, "Okay, I'm here whenever" in that carefree way of hers. She brought so much lightness to my transition, and to my life, and I'm positive that if I hadn't seen how effortlessly open she was on YouTube, I wouldn't have shared as much as I did on *Drag Race.* In the eyes of Gigi Gorgeous, life is beautiful and fun. It's the best vibe ever.

Contributors

These are our gorgeous friends and family who shared their stories with us—and with you. We thank them all for contributing.

 ADAM LAMBERT • Adam Lambert is a recording artist and actor. Runner-up on season 8 of *American Idol*, Lambert has released four solo studio albums and toured and performed with Queen. He has appeared in *Bohemian Rhapsody, Glee,* and *The Rocky Horror Picture Show: Let's Do the Time Warp Again*, among other productions.

 ALOK • ALOK is a writer, performance artist, and media personality. They are a mixed-media artist, using poetry, comedy, fashion design, social media, and more, to explore themes of gender, race, trauma, and the human condition.

 AMANDA LEPORE • Amanda Lepore is a model, singer, and performance artist. A former Club Kid, she has appeared in advertising for numerous companies. A regular subject of David LaChapelle, she has also worked with photographers Ruben van Schalm and Terry Richardson, among others.

 CANDIS CAYNE • Acting since the age of 10, Candis Cayne made history as the first transgender actress to play a recurring role on primetime network television in *Dirty Sexy Money*. She has also appeared on *Drop Dead Diva, RuPaul's Drag Race, The Magicians,* and *Grey's Anatomy*. She has collaborated with GLAAD and the Human Rights Campaign, and authored , *Hi, Gorgeous!: Transforming Inner Power into Radiant Beauty*.

 COURTNEY ACT • Courtney Act is a drag queen, singer, author, and television personality. She first came to prominence competing on the first season of *Australian Idol*. Most notably, she appeared on season 6 of *RuPaul's Drag Race*, finishing as a runner-up. Her memoir, *Caught in the Act*, was published in 2022.

 JAMIE RAINES • Jamie Raines is a YouTube personality and LGBTQ+ advocate. His content includes commentary on gender identity and LGBTQ+ issues, as well as general lifestyle topics. He documented his gender transition, including the effects of hormone replacement therapy and gender-affirming surgery, on his channel, Jammidodger.

 JAZZ JENNINGS • Jazz Jennings is a YouTube personality, spokesmodel, television personality, and LGBTQ+ rights activist. One of the youngest publicly documented people to be identified as transgender, Jennings is a cofounder of the TransKids Purple Rainbow Foundation, which assists trans youth. She stars in the TLC reality series *I Am Jazz*, which focuses on her personal and family life as a teen and young adult.

LA DEMI MARTINEZ • La Demi Martinez is a reality television and social media personality. Having appeared in *Ex on the Beach* and *The Love Boat*, among other productions, La Demi fights against society's manufactured gender identification and labeling.

 LAITH ASHLEY • Laith Ashley is a model, actor, activist, and entertainer. He has appeared in *Strut*, *RuPaul's Drag Race*, and *Pose*, and had modeled for *GQ*, *Vogue*, *OUT*, *Attitude*, and *Gay Times*, among others.

 LINA BRADFORD • Lina Bradford is a DJ born, raised, and based in New York City. She identified as trans at a young age and began her entertainment career as a dancer. Having performed with several companies around the city for 11 years, she now incorporates those moves into her signature DJ style.

 NATS GETTY • Nats Getty is a model, designer, and LGBTQ+ rights activist. He is the brand owner of the fashion house Strike Oil, works closely with GLAAD, and is an adviser to the Ariadne Getty Foundation. He is married to Gigi Gorgeous.

 PARIS HILTON • Paris Hilton is an entrepreneur, influencer, reality television personality, and much more. After starring in *The Simple Life*, she built an empire as a DJ, actress, model, author, and recording artist, among others. She is the subject of the documentary *This Is Paris* and hosts the podcast of the same name.

 SARAH McBRIDE • Sarah McBride is a politician and activist. A Democratic member of the Delaware senate since January 2021, she is the first openly transgender elected official in U.S. history. She was previously the National Press Secretary for the Human Rights Campaign. Her book, *Tomorrow Will Be Different: Love, Loss, and the Fight for Trans Equality*, was published in 2018.

 SASHA COLBY • Sasha Colby is a drag performer and actor who holds the title of Miss Continental 2012. She competed on season 15 of *RuPaul's Drag Race* and has appeared in television shows such as *Hawaii Five-0* and *Boss'd Up*, along with several music videos.

 SCHUYLER BAILAR • Schuyler Bailar is a swimmer and the first openly transgender athlete to compete in an NCAA D1 sport as a man. His first middle-grade novel, *Obie Is Man Enough*, was published in 2021.

 TIFFANY NAMTU • The sister of Gigi Gorgeous, Tiffany Namtu is a recording artist who has contributed to songs and podcasts, as well as an advocate for the Ariadne Getty Foundation. She can be found on Instagram at @tiffaneyney.

 VIOLET CHACHKI • Violet Chachki is the winner of *RuPaul's Drag Race* season 7 and one of the world's leading drag superstars. She is a recording artist, burlesque performer, aerialist, model, and co-host of "No Gorge," a podcast and YouTube show, alongside Gottmik. Violet is the first drag queen ever to attend the prestigious Met Gala and has appeared in fashion campaigns for Prada, Moschino, and Jean Paul Gaultier. She has also performed in several music videos for artists such as Beyonce, Sam Smith, Kim Petras, and Allie X, among others.

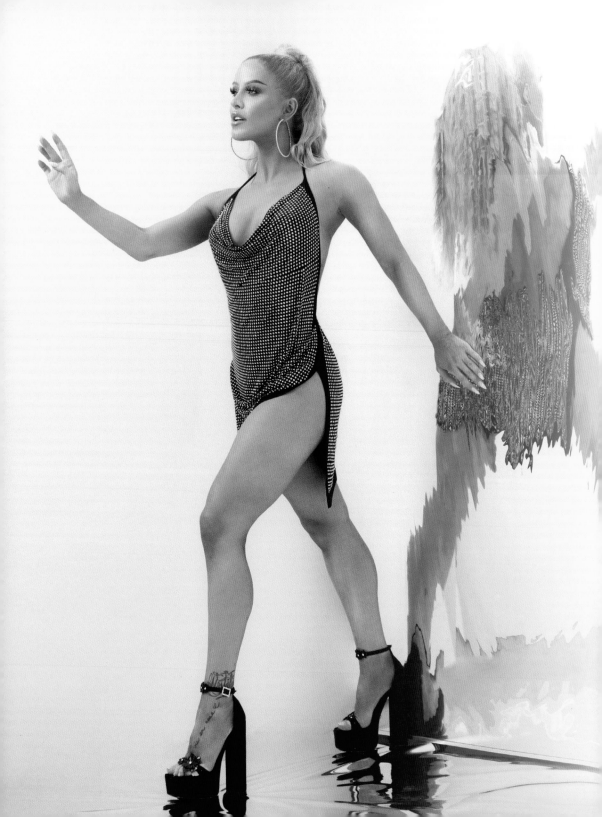

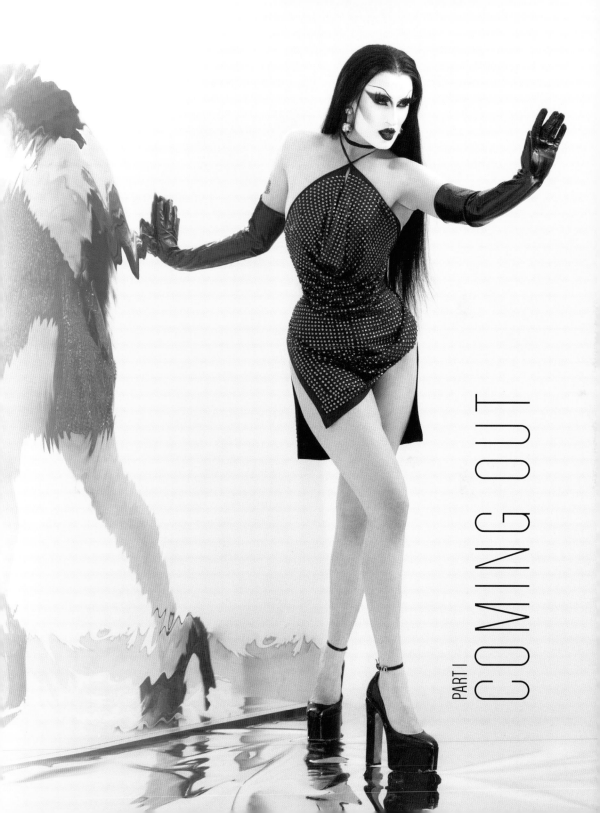

PART I COMING OUT

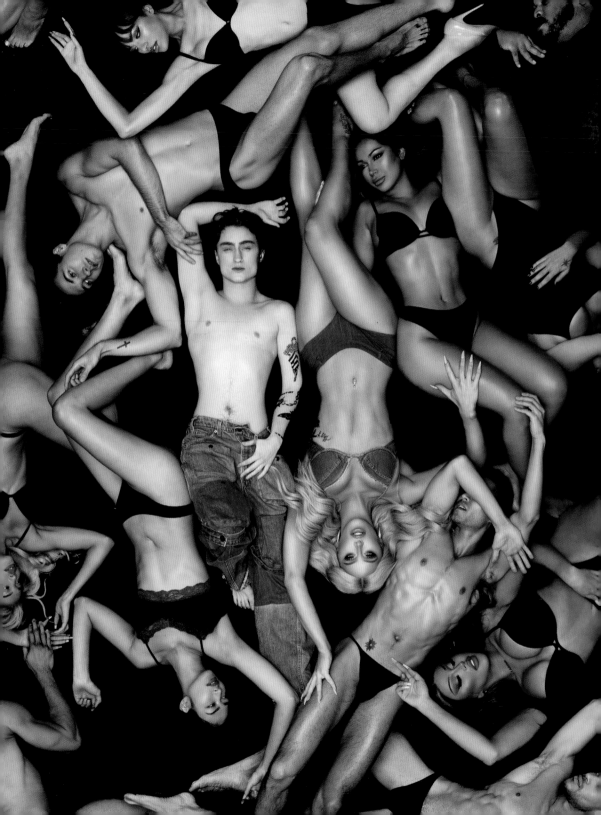

Gender & Sex

People often get these words confused, but they're definitely not the same thing. A person's gender is defined by how they see themselves, and a person's sex is usually assigned by whatever their genitals look like at birth, but this is complicated. We all have lots of different sexual characteristics, many of which change during our lifetimes. Intersex people, for example, have characteristics that do not fit into the binary idea of strictly male or female.

GOTTMIK: Gender is up here [points to head] and sexuality is down here [points to nether region].

GIGI: Gender's who I am. Sexuality is who I love.

GOTTMIK: Gender is a social construct.

GIGI: And it's a journey. Every stage of my transition has come with a new level of acceptance. In the beginning, I felt more of a need to do girl stuff only. Then later, I dropped that. Now I'm like, *I can have some stereotypical manly traits, too. It's fine.* I don't have to be all girl all the time. The parts of myself that a lot of people would consider to be masculine qualities, like my loudness and my dominance, are part of me, too.

GOTTMIK: What's interesting is that loudness and dominance are considered to be masculine traits. Who made that up? I have to constantly check in with myself to make sure I'm making choices because I want to, and not because of the pressure I'm getting from society. When I think about bottom surgery, it's like, *Yeah, I want that.* And then I'm like, *But why do I want that? Do I want that for the right reasons? Is it something that I need, or am I letting society define what it means to be a man?*

GIGI: Right. You have to check in with yourself. Everybody's journey is so personal, and the spectrum of gender and sexuality is nuanced. You can be a trans man or a trans woman and still have traits of the opposite gender.

GOTTMIK: Yes. I personally love presenting as masculine, but if I have little feminine moments, I'm okay with that.

GIGI: I have a Barbie aesthetic, and a lot of people ask me if that's partly because there's pressure in the trans female community to be hyper girly. I've felt some societal pressure for sure, but a lot of my pressure has been self-imposed. Now, I'm more relaxed about how I present, because I feel more relaxed within myself. I can be loud and domineering sometimes and sweet and passive other times. I feel welcoming of all these characteristics now.

GOTTMIK: My friend, Violet, is a great example of someone who doesn't subscribe to society's ideas about gender. One day she'll wake up and be like, "I'm a girl today," and another day, she'll wake up and be somewhere on the spectrum between girl and boy. She doesn't feel the need to transition. She's just very cool with who she is, and how people perceive her doesn't affect her mentally in any way. It's amazing.

GIGI: I think that's a good reminder that there are so many ways to define what gender and sexuality mean to you. If it feels right to you, then it's perfect.

GOTTMIK: Right, whatever you decide to do is perfect, and in the meantime, the world around you is going to continue to be imperfect.

Here's an example: there's this sex toy company that divides the products on their website into two sections: one for men and one for women. And I'm like, *Hello, sex is not gender!*

GIGI: Do they know there are chicks with dicks out there?

GOTTMIK: Apparently not. It's just makes trans people feel excluded. Why not organize that differently? Why the two sections?

GIGI: So easy to fix.

GOTTMIK: But a lot of cis hetero people aren't considering the trans experience.

GIGI: Right. That type of stuff can be super triggering in the beginning, and then over time you learn to have a sense of humor about it. Getting misgendered, too, is another source of major discomfort when you're first starting out, or at least it was for me. Can I tell you a story about a forehead vein in Orange County?

GOTTMIK: Please.

GIGI: I went to see a doctor in Orange County to have a vein removed from my forehead. In order for him to see it more clearly, I had to sit upside down in a medical chair so it would protrude. Such awkward positioning. Such *vulnerable* positioning! There I was, sitting upside down in a T-shirt and leggings, and this doctor said to the nurse, "Will you put his legs up?" I was like, *Um, what? Is he talking about me?* I was the only person in the room besides the nurse, so clearly he was talking about me. The nurse took the order and put my legs up, and I was just hanging out there, upside down, thinking, *How did I just get misgendered?* I ran my palm over my chin. Was it stubbly? I didn't think it was that stubbly. Afterward, my friend picked me up and I told her what had happened. "I just got misgendered," I said, and she replied, "I mean, we are in Orange County." Then we laughed about it. You can't let that type of stuff ruin your day.

GOTTMIK: Yes. Even if you're comfortable with who you are, when you get misgendered, you instantly think, *What am I giving right now? Why am I feminine to them? Why am I masculine to them?* You go into this spiral, but hopefully not for too long. And then you just have to laugh, because a lot of the time, it means nothing. My cisgender male friends get called "ma'am" sometimes. It just happens.

GIGI: After I got my boobs, I didn't think anybody was going to misgender me. I wore a push-up bra and the sluttiest clothes to avoid it. That was 10 years ago, when the world was very different. Now we're all asking each other what pronouns we use.

GOTTMIK: Right? We've come so far. And we still have so far to go.

Find Yourself

with Courtney Act

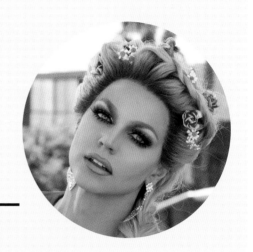

PHOTO BY **MITCH FONG**

I never felt like I fit into the world, and I always wondered if that was because I was trans.

I started drag when I was 18, and I looked so femme and felt so comfortable as Courtney. I loved being a girl. I didn't feel like a man, so, by process of elimination, I realized that I must be a woman. Those were the only options back then.

But I loved being a boy, too. It felt to me like something was broken. Was it me?

When the terms *gender fluid* and *gender nonconforming* became more popular, I came to the conclusion that it was okay for boys to be feminine and girls to be masculine. I found comfort in these terms. They fit me. I had been trying to make myself fit into the rules of the broken world, when I thought I was the broken one.

Was I mad that nobody explained this to me earlier? Yeah, but now I know who I am because I had to come to understand myself outside of the status quo. I became myself, and that's powerful. I stand so strong now in who I am and feel such peace and joy around my gender, sexuality, and identity. I actually think that not fitting in turned out to be my greatest teacher.

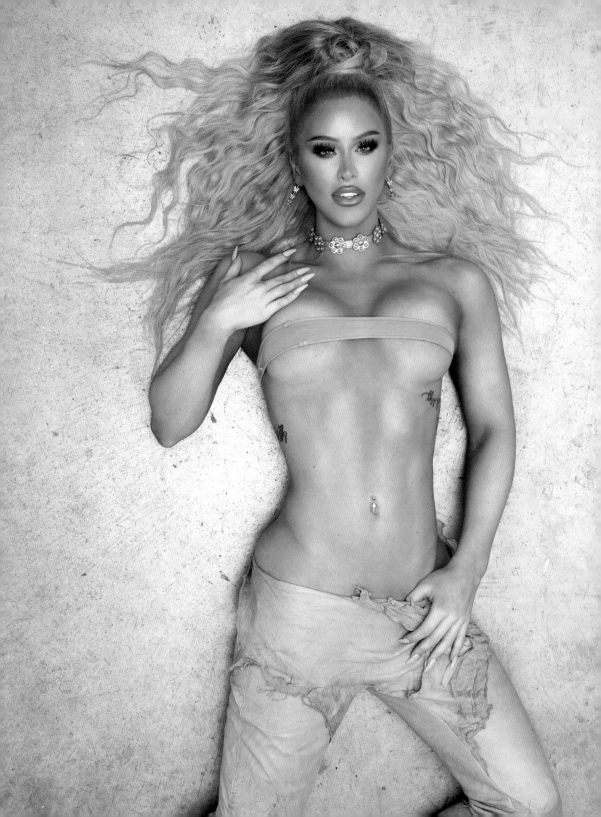

Deciding to Come Out

Most people, before they actually come out, spend time wondering about it. *Is this right for me? Is it not?* The only person who can really answer those questions is you. After you do decide to come out, the next step is figuring out who to tell first. Unfortunately, some friends and family members might not react in the way that you want, which is why it's super important to have a strong queer support group.

GOTTMIK: I like to be sure of what I think before I start talking about it, and sometimes I need to think about something for a really long time. I spent years thinking, *I'm pretty sure I'm trans*, but I didn't come out, because part of me was hoping I could slide by as a more masculine girl. Transitioning is not a fun little walk in the park. It's really hard. It got to a point where I was waking up crying every day. So finally, I decided, *Okay, this has to change.* And I told Gigi Gorgeous and Nats Getty, who I am so insanely blessed are my best friends because they understand me so well.

GIGI: For me, it was different. I was really gung ho about coming out—four times! I came out as gay when I was 15 or 16. Then I came out as trans when I was 19. I came out as a lesbian when I was 24 or 25. And then I came out as pansexual, meaning I could be attracted to anyone, regardless of their identity, when I was 28. I think a lot of people feel like it's a huge hurdle, especially coming out as trans, because it's such a lifestyle change. But for a lot of people, once they get to the other side, it's fucking epic. If thinking about coming out is keeping you up at night, then something's got to change. You have to either get into it or get lost, because nobody's going to make the change but you.

GOTTMIK: Yeah, if you're not happy, then whatever you're doing isn't working. For a long time, I didn't even know why I was unhappy. Was it because I thought I might be trans and I didn't know how to deal with it? Or was it because I was just depressed? The first step was figuring out the answers to those questions. After I finally realized that I was sad because I was trans and I hadn't admitted it to myself yet, I was like, *Okay, what do I do next?* I had to accept it before I could move forward.

GIGI: And accepting it is a lot easier said than done, of course. If your situation makes it hard to come out, like for example if you're young and living at home and too scared to be honest with the people around you, or if you're just not sure about what you want to say yet, then try to keep yourself happy until you have your answers. I know that might sound trite, but it can be useful. Go running if you love running. Do anything that releases your serotonin. If you're in the limbo space between thinking about coming out and actually doing it, it can be so easy to spiral.

GOTTMIK: Yeah, and I think protecting your energy is so important, too. When I was first transitioning I literally did not even want to talk to a straight person or I would get pissed. I didn't want to deal with getting misgendered. I didn't want any questions. I just wanted to have fun. Now I look back on that and I can see that it was an instinctual self-protection thing.

GIGI: Would you say you were more insecure back then?

GOTTMIK: Oh my God, yeah. I just could not handle the comments.

GIGI: For me, it's a day-to-day thing, too. Some days, I'm definitely more sensitive. I can feel the comments coming and I'm like, *Oh no, this is not a good vibe*. Other days, I don't care. But I do think that in the beginning, it's so important to guard your energy because it's easier to get triggered.

GOTTMIK: Yes. That's a big fear with coming out. You're worried about how other people are going to perceive you. Even now, I'm sometimes so bothered if I get a weird comment. It really depends on the day, though. Sometimes, I can shake it off, and other times, I'm like, *I have to go home*.

GIGI: Yes! Like bothered. Day ruined. It's so up and down.

GOTTMIK: Right. And on the subject of appearances, I think one of the reasons I didn't transition for so long was because I didn't see a lot of examples of men I wanted to look like. Every trans guy I saw in the media was hyper-masculine and muscle-obsessed. When I moved to LA and finally met trans guys who didn't look like that, I was finally able to say, "Oh, I want this." That's when I officially decided I was trans.

GIGI: I officially decided when I met a trans girl named Betty in New York. I was 19. I'll tell you a little more about her later, but basically, seeing how she lived made me realize that I wanted to live in the same way.

GOTTMIK: Coming out is so much easier if you know people who have what you want.

GIGI: Absolutely. Now, when I look back at myself at that age, it's funny to me that it wasn't totally obvious to me that I was trans. Because in my childhood, there were so many clues. When I was really young, for example, like before the age when I understood what shame was, I made my brothers call me Kim. I have no idea where I got that name, because this was pre–Kim Kardashian, clearly, but my brothers were happy to go along with it. That was the first time I thought, *I'm a girl*.

GOTTMIK: Same. Looking back, there were so many signs for me, too. I wore the boy's uniforms at school; I wanted the boy's toys at McDonald's; I was the only girl at the all-boys party. I'd look around at the other girls and be like, *We are not the same*. I think I wanted top surgery before I even fully knew what it was. And my dad caught me peeing standing up once. After I transitioned, my parents told me they almost took me to therapy when I was young because I never had any girlfriends growing up.

GIGI: I used to put a towel on my head and pretend that it was hair. And I remember when I was in my early 20s, I heard this trans girl's mom say that she found her daughter in the bathroom trying to cut her penis off. And I had full-on flashback of keeping scissors in the bathroom when I was young. I never tried to do it. But I was thinking about doing it.

GOTTMIK: I personally wish my parents had put me on hormone blockers, so I always assumed if I had a child expressing they were trans I would immediately put them on blockers, but after doing some research I've learned that it is not that easy of a decision. Hormone blockers are very serious and require a lot of research prior to usage. So if you're a parent reading this, my advice would be to listen to your child, really do your research, and talk to doctors who know how to administer them safely. There are so many different sides and outcomes that can weigh in on the final decision. But at the end of the day, making sure you're supporting your child and making sure they're happy is the most important thing.

GIGI: Right. There are so many options now that didn't exist when we were growing up. And I think the bigger takeaway is about support. If you have support from your friends and family, it's a million times easier to come out.

GOTTMIK: And after you come out to family and friends, there's the question of who else you're going to come out to.

GIGI: Exactly. I knew I wanted to be as honest as possible with as many people as possible. That's why I started sharing my life online. What was amazing about that was how much positive feedback I received from all these strangers who I never would have met walking down the street in Canada. Of course, I got negative feedback, too, but I focused on the positive. Posts that said, "You look so pretty," or "You look happy now" made me feel so good. My supporters became my backbone.

I'd been on hormones for a few months before I finally decided to come out as trans publicly. And when I did it, people were so proud of me. I'd had no surgery, no name change. I had no idea what I was doing. I was just like, "This is about to be a journey for all of us." I feel like people I hadn't even met became my chosen family.

Also, sharing online in that way felt really safe to me, because I was making these videos alone in my bedroom. Nobody could speak back to me. It's kind of like you, Gottmik, doing your confessionals on *Drag Race*. They're edited down to show the best moments. That's how I edited my videos, too.

GOTTMIK: Right, yes. It's very comfortable and controlled when there's editing involved.

GIGI: It was real life, but the best versions of our real lives.

GOTTMIK: I met someone recently who has a Finsta [fake, or private, Instagram account]. She has zero followers and thousands of posts. She started it as a kind of diary about her transition, which I think is amazing.

GIGI: It's so important to be open about how you're feeling. Whether it's to one person, to a camera, to a Finsta, or to a journal. The first part of coming out is about being honest with yourself, and the next part is about being honest with other people. It's scary, but once you come out publicly, the coolest things can happen. You never know what kind of impact you're going to have by sharing your truth. You could change the course of somebody's life.

GOTTMIK: What are some of the other things that made you feel better when you were in the beginning of your transition?

GIGI: Music. When I first came out, I listened to a lot of Gaga. Music is just a really easy way to change your mood. When I'm feeling down, I love to blast my favorite songs.

GOTTMIK: Yeah, music does help. Before *Drag Race*, I listened to this artist named Ben Platt, who I love so much. A lot of his songs are about what it's like to live and to love as a gay guy in society. I used to have this routine of waking up every morning and stretching and listening to Ben Platt. And it really did help me, now that I think back on it. Recently, we became friends online. But he has no idea yet how deep my fandom goes.

GIGI: You should tell him! Another thing that has always lightened my mood is makeup. When I look good, I feel better. It's as simple as that.

GOTTMIK: I've had some experience with therapy, too. That's been majorly helpful to a lot of people I know.

GIGI: As with everything else, the answer is to figure out what works for you. You're a unique snowflake, and your journey is not going to look exactly like anybody else's.

Adam Lambert *on*
Coming Out

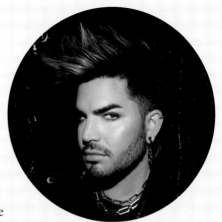

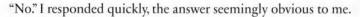

PHOTO BY **JOSEPH SINCLAIR**

When I was 18, I was outed by my mother and it was a relief. While I was driving us home after an event, she asked me quite simply, "Do you have a girlfriend?"

"No." I responded quickly, the answer seemingly obvious to me.

"Would you like one?"

I hesitated, knowing where this was going. "Um, no?"

There was a pregnant pause, sweat starting to bead on my upper lip. I wasn't sure if she was going to leave it at that, or—

"Well, do you have a boyfriend?" Her voice climbed to a higher register.

Matching her pitch, I said "Nooo."

Another pause. "Would you like one?"

This was it. My official statement of intent. My closet being thrown open with a nearly breathless response. "Yes?"

Whew! This was what I'd been building up to for years, never being sure of how it would be received.

I glanced over at my smiling mother, who replied, "Finally!"

We both laughed. It turned out that many years prior to that night, my mother had visited the San Diego LGBT center, asking how to best support a closeted child. She was advised to wait until I was ready to come to her. She followed the advice for a few years before instinctively knowing it was okay to ask. All I needed was a gentle nudge. Mothers always know.

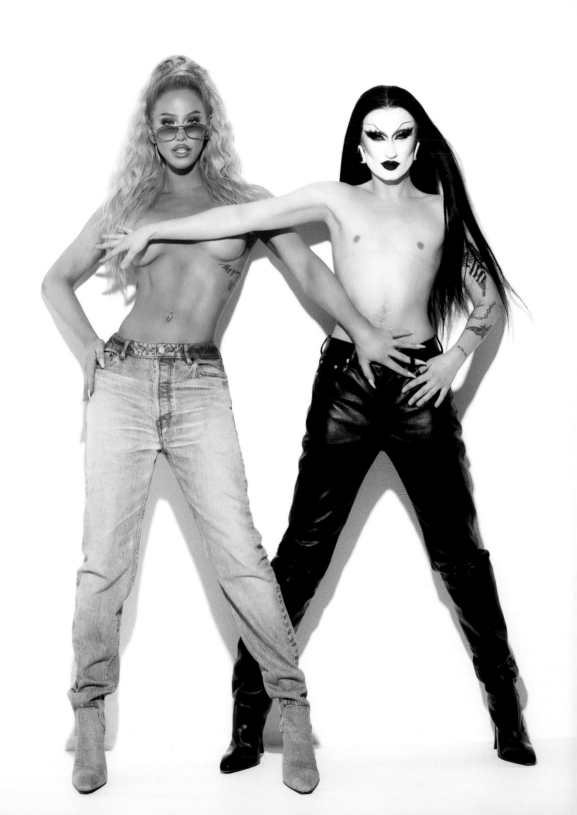

Choosing a Name

These are the most important things to know: (a) your name should feel like you and (b) if you need to change your name again later, it's fine. As far as the legal logistics, each U.S. state has different rules, so make sure you look up what's required of you in order to change your name and/or your gender on your state-issued ID. Some states are super lax about gender, and others (at least at the time of this writing) require proof of complete gender reassignment surgery, which is just medieval.

GIGI: Here's how I got my name: My mom thought I was going to be a girl when I was still cooking inside of her. She was going to name me Lauren. I always loved that, so I chose it as my middle name, but I changed the spelling. I made it Loren, as in Sophia Loren. I had a poster of her in my room when I was young, and I was obsessed with how pretty she was. My first name came from my old online name, Gregory Gorgeous, which people would often abbreviate as G. G. So when it came time to picking a name, Gigi already felt natural to me.

If I'd had a unisex name, though, I definitely wouldn't have changed it. There's this trans girl on TikTok who is taking everyone along with her on her trans journey. Her name is Dylan Mulvaney, which is her birth name. She chose to keep it. I think it's so dope. If you have a unisex name, then you don't have to go through the whole process of asking people to relearn your name if you don't want to. You just change your pronouns. Which is so much less triggering.

GOTTMIK: I have two name change stories, one for my drag name and one for my name-name. I'll tell you the drag name one first: I grew up with four Mikaylas on my soccer team, so we all changed our names. I ended up being G, because my last name's Gottlieb. My parents sometimes still call me G. I liked the idea of mixing up pieces of my old names, because it just felt familiar to me. So I paired the "Mik" of Mikayla with the "Gott" of Gottlieb. In high school, I made Gottmik my Instagram handle and I put it on my license plate. It's framed and hanging on my wall at home right now.

After I realized I was trans, I had to choose a name-name, which happened pretty organically. One day, I was watching porn and the star's name was Kade. The K sound was familiar, because it's in the name Mikayla.

What I would say to people who are trying to choose a name is just have fun with it.

GIGI: Yes! It's so fun choosing a name. Once you find the right one, you'll know. It will just sound right to you.

GOTTMIK: And don't feel like you have to commit to your first choice. There's so much pressure put on the name change thing, but it's really not necessary. I know people who've chosen a bunch of new names before landing on the right one.

GIGI: And it's not like you have to legally change your name and gender on day one. I don't think that's recommended anyway. Give it some time.

GOTTMIK: Yeah, making the legal changes is tedious. And it can be expensive, depending on where you are.

GIGI: I don't think changing my name was expensive in Canada, at least not 10 years ago when I did it. But I do remember they asked me tons of questions. "Why are you changing your name? Are you getting married?" I had to provide a letter from a psychiatrist, too. It was uncomfortable. I was like, "Why do I have to prove myself to you?"

GOTTMIK: The process is the worst. When I finally got my new ID in the mail, though, it was so validating.

GIGI: Oh my God, same. And even though mine still said "male" for a little bit, I would just hand it over at the airport or whatever and hope they didn't check the gender. Once Nats was booking me a flight and he asked me to send him a picture of my passport, so I did, but I covered the gender with my nail. Obviously, he knew I was trans, but just that little letter was so triggering.

GOTTMIK: California's amazing with the gender change. You just go to the DMV and tell them your gender.

GIGI: Yeah, Canada's gotten their shit together on that front, too. You just fill out one simple form. So easy. And I'm so glad I'm not getting my dead name called out at the airport anymore. Every time that happened, I'd be like, *Is God trying to test me?*

GOTTMIK: That's happened to me, too.

GIGI: I'd wait a beat before going up to the front desk, but after my ID said, "Gigi, female," I was like, *I'm unstoppable, bitch.*

GOTTMIK: It's so freeing when the name has been chosen and it's official.

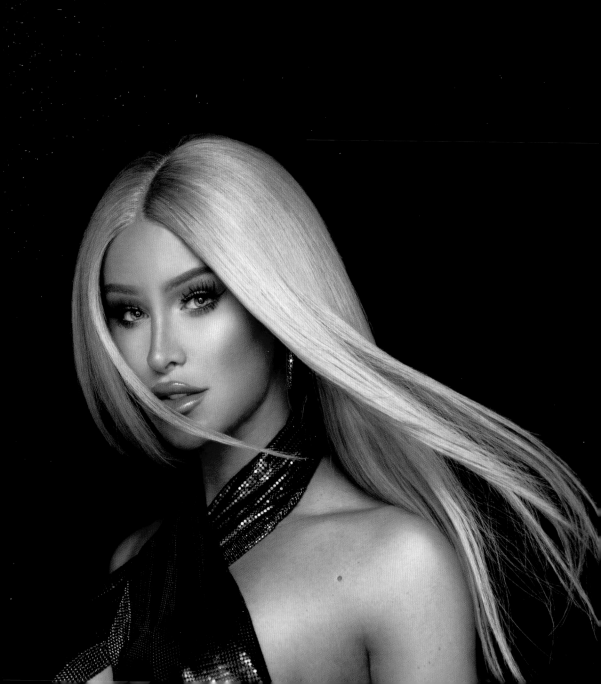

Advice for Parents

Parents, if your kid comes out to you, the only correct response is, "I love you." Even if you're freaking out inside, still say, "I love you." And after that, just listen to what your kid is telling you. If you don't know anything about being trans, then start educating yourself. Read books; watch videos online; meet with gender specialists. If you're reading this book, then you're already on the right track.

GOTTMIK: My parents are very conservative. They knew nothing about queer people. When I was 15 and they found out I went to Pride, they literally cried. So obviously they thought me being trans was the end of the world. They also thought it was a phase, and that I'd moved to LA and been indoctrinated by strange people. I was so over them. I hated their reaction, and I was ready to cut them off. Then you invited them to LA, Gigi, and after that trip, they realized it wasn't a phase, and they got into acceptance.

GIGI: I feel a huge thing I learned is that transitioning is a transition for you and for everyone around you. Because a lot of people are confused about what it means to be trans, that means that you kind of automatically become an educator.

GOTTMIK: Obviously, if your parents are unsafe or too unloving to bear, then maybe not talking to them for a while is the right thing to do. That wasn't the right thing to do with my parents. I actually learned that I needed to be more patient with them. They just cried a lot, and I interpreted that as them being unsupportive, but that was wrong. They weren't unsupportive. They were just confused.

GIGI: I lost my mom when I was 19, before I came out as trans. Later that same year, I came out to my dad, who, like your parents, is really conservative. I would say that he was confused, too, but he dealt with his confusion in a quiet way. He didn't cry. We didn't get into screaming matches. But even despite his lack of emotion, I could tell he wasn't into it. He would misgender me a lot and dead-name me. I found it so frustrating. Sometimes, it would make me angry and I'd say, "I'm not telling you anything anymore!"

Now, I see that I could have been so much nicer to my dad. He just didn't get it, and I didn't fully understand at that point that him not getting it was normal! He didn't know any trans people. Why would I expect him to understand? I wish I'd educated him a little more instead of getting mad.

GOTTMIK: I so agree, but I also think you have to strike a balance with the educating as a queer person. When it's someone who's really important to you, like your parents, of course you're going to educate them if they seem open to it. But it's not your responsibility to educate everyone in the world. You have to be in a place where you feel emotionally, spiritually, and mentally capable of educating in order to do it well. And if you're not in that place, then it's okay. I feel most compelled to educate someone when they seem really open to it.

GIGI: Which brings us to our advice for parents: be open, parents!

GOTTMIK: Yes. Try to be a good listener, and take the initiative to educate yourself. Buy books; watch documentaries. No matter what, you should just let your kid be themselves and try to guide them in the best way you know how. Because that's what you signed up for as a parent.

GIGI: Exactly. Every loving parent says that same thing. They want their kid to be happy and successful, right? When I came out as gay to my parents (which was after I saw Adam Lambert on *American Idol*, by the way), my mom cried. She was sad because she thought my life was going to be harder, and she worried that I wouldn't be successful. So, become successful, people! And that doesn't necessarily mean getting money or fame. It just means thriving.

GOTTMIK: Right, you can define success in whatever way feels right to you. If you're thriving, then when you come out to your parents, it will be harder for them to be worried about how your life is going to suck because you're trans. After my parents saw how much happier I was as a trans guy, and how much more comfortable I was in my body, they were happy for me. Just being happy is a success. And surrounding yourself with people who accept you is a success, too.

GIGI: A lot of parents' knee-jerk reaction is to say, "This is a phase." Because they're uncomfortable. Don't do this, parents! Don't disagree with whatever your kid is telling you. If you want to be in their life, then get into it. Otherwise, you can get lost.

GOTTMIK: "Get into it or get lost!" I literally said that to my parents when they were crying. And then after they got into it my dad joined a PFLAG group.

GIGI: What's PFLAG?

GOTTMIK: Parents, Families, and Friends of Lesbians and Gays. The fact that my dad was really trying was so cute to me. Put in some effort, parents. Show your kid you love them.

GIGI: I feel one popular mistake parents make is thinking that they've failed in some way, and wondering what they're going to tell their friends. This type of selfishness is so not useful. If your kid comes out to you, don't think about yourself. Think about your kid.

GOTTMIK: I have two uncles who won't even talk to me anymore. So, my parents cut off contact with them. My mom doesn't go to her brother's house anymore. I think that's a good example of a selfless parent. And it's a good example of how this has been a transition for them, too.

GIGI: Can you imagine coming out to your parents and them not protecting you like that? It's such a vulnerable thing to share. Sharing it is an act of trust.

GOTTMIK: The least you can do, parents, is say, "I love you." And then start your education process with Google.

GIGI: Get into it or get lost, parents! That's the Gigi/Gottmik method.

A Mother's Pause

with **Tiffany Namtu**

PHOTO BY **GIGI GORGEOUS GETTY**

My biggest fear was that my mom would never look at me in the same way after coming out to her. In Canada, where we both live, we don't know a lot of queer people. Gigi is the first trans person I ever met. I started going to LA a lot to visit her, and that's when I got exposed to a community that was the opposite of the one I have in Canada. Pretty much everyone I hang out with in LA is queer. So, I had all this exposure to queer life, whereas my mom had basically none.

At the age of 31, when I came out to her as pan, she was shocked. She said, "I love you," and then she told me that she needed to think about it for a minute. She said she had to gather her thoughts. I was devastated. That definitely wasn't the perfect reaction I had wanted, and it confirmed my worst fear. She was never going to look at me in the same way again.

Thankfully, I ended up being wrong about that. After getting over her shock, she moved into acceptance. Looking back, I can see that she needed to go through her own process of absorbing the information and coming to terms with it, which was exactly what I had needed to do when I first realized I was pan. Now, I don't think it was such a bad thing that she asked for a pause. It was just honest. She needed time. Coming out is a process for everyone, it turns out.

If I could do it all over again, I might not spend as much time psyching myself out beforehand. When you come out to someone, they're either going to accept you or they're not. And even though it feels better to be accepted by the people you love, acceptance isn't really the goal. The goal is for you to feel free.

My Journey with Gigi

by **David Lazzarato**

PHOTO COURTESY **DAVID LAZZARATO** AND **LORI LOPARCO**

In order to share my perspectives as Gigi's father, I have to begin with some background to properly set the context. Prior to her transitioning, Greg was an outgoing, energetic, and decisive guy who excelled at everything he set his mind to. He was the middle child of three boys, and my wife, Judy, and I were proud of him and his brothers, Adam and Cory. Greg inherited the outgoing trait from his mom. While I am not an introvert, I am a bit more on the conservative side.

In 2008, at the age of 16, Greg told his mom and I he was gay. We were surprised but not shocked, I guess, because he did not hide his more feminine characteristics or behaviors (e.g., choices of clothes, use of makeup, etc.). We both thought that Greg was a very expressive individual and those choices were part of that side of him. Our reaction was to accept what he told us and focus on our concern for his happiness and safety. Judy passed away early in 2012 after battling cancer for four years. Her passing was a painful and huge loss to everyone who knew her, especially to me and our three boys. At that point, I was a single parent and knew I needed to somehow fill both roles for all my kids.

It was November 2013 when Greg told me, "Dad, I am not gay. I am transgender." I thought for a few seconds (which felt like an eternity) and asked "What do you mean by transgender?" I thought I knew what she meant, but it was the only thing I could think of saying in that moment. "I am a woman trapped in a man's body, and I plan to do everything I can to change that. From now on, my name is Gigi." At that moment, I was uncertain about what would happen next. What could or should I do to help her? How would family and friends react? I was fearful for Gigi's long-term happiness and safety. I just remember telling her I loved her, her mother loved her from above, and her brothers and family loved her, before giving her a big hug.

Gigi had done her homework long before telling me of her decision. She had talked to friends (including transgender ones) and doctors and was moving forward with or without my approval or involvement, as she had already started estrogen injections. She was also an online YouTube personality at this point and decided she was going to be very open about her decision with the people who followed her. There was never a thought to try to change her mind. That would have driven a wedge between us that I didn't want. Instead, I tried to stay close and understand as much as I could about what might be ahead of us.

I initially wondered how family and friends would react, but Gigi's expectation was that everyone would understand and respect her decision immediately, and that we would all get the she/her pronouns right all the time. Well, I didn't do so well on that front, and it took Gigi a long time to appreciate that I could be supportive of her decision even though I didn't always use the right name or pronouns. Twenty years of using "Greg" and he/him pronouns didn't make the change easy to adapt to quickly for me. It took a while, but I realized I was mourning the loss of my son as I was trying to figure out how to build a relationship with my new daughter.

Family and friends were an important source of support for me throughout Gigi's transition. I started to tell them of Gigi's decision and plans before I fully understood them, and I would say they had one of three reactions. First, the majority of them were supportive but admitted they didn't know a lot about transitioning. Second, some were supportive and told me of friends or neighbors who were going through similar transitions with a family member. Third, some listened quietly and didn't say much, which was all right, too. But the caring and love from all of them enabled me to continue to have an open mind and be close to Gigi throughout her journey.

One of the friends I relied upon the most was a woman named Lori, whom I had worked with years earlier and had begun seeing in 2013. Lori and Gigi have gotten to know each other very well since then because Lori and I got married in 2015! Lori wanted to help Gigi and me in any way she could. She was conscious not to overstep and really worked at building a relationship between adult women, and not one that would at all feel like she was trying to replace Gigi's mom. Between the two of us, we now have six adult children with more than enough love and support to go around. Thank you Lori, and *Ti amo per sempre!*

It was obvious that Gigi didn't need help with her day-to-day decisions or actions. In fact, I was probably not high on her list of people to ask for that type of advice. But when she told me of her plans to have facial surgery and breast implants, we had several long conversations about the pros and cons. I was very concerned, to say the least. She explained she was only going to use extremely experienced doctors for the surgeries, and I took some comfort in that. She also said "Don't worry, Dad, friends will be with me when I do this," and I told her I would be there as well and it wasn't open for debate. I have never felt closer to Gigi than I did being with her during those recovery periods!

I have often thought about what I could have done differently. Looking back, I should have found an experienced counselor to talk to during the beginning of the process and onward—someone I could share the worries and fears with that I didn't feel comfortable talking to others about. I often use the expression "can't hurt, might help" when talking about whether to do different things. On this point, I would recommend parents do as I say, not as I did!

Being transgender is a journey, not a specific event. The personality of the individual does not change in that process, but how they present themselves to the world changes and evolves. Parents, family, and friends have a decision to make early on. Do they want to figure out how to be supportive, or do they want to let their views and experiences get in the way of the person's decisions and happiness? It is a conscious choice that has to be made, and I would recommend it be made very early in the transitioning journey. As people consider what they are going to do, please think back and remember all the times your parents, family, or the closest of friends disagreed with some of your important choices and decisions and how that made you feel.

It has been almost 10 years now, and Gigi is extremely happy and I respect her for the decisions she made and for the perseverance required to do what she wanted. I am also very proud of her willingness to spend time and share her experiences with people wrestling with the tough decisions she faced.

Gigi, know we all love you, and your mom would be so proud of you!

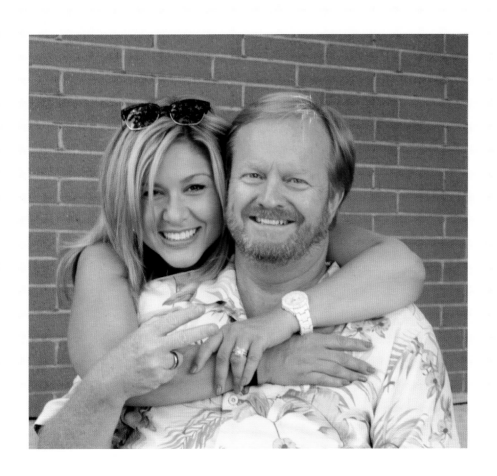

The "Right" Way

by **Robert Gottlieb**

One day, every parent transitions to life with children without an instruction manual. We all struggle to raise our children the best we can with the resources we have and the knowledge we've acquired through our journeys in life, convinced that we're doing it "right." But in the process, we sometimes forget that our children are their own individuals, just like us.

When we first learned of Kade's transgender identity, we admittedly struggled with it, and there were lots of tears and fears. For a conservative, Christian family, learning the truth was not easy. We knew so little of what it meant to be transgender. Communication and understanding are key at a time when parents know little about this topic and even the child is learning to express themselves authentically.

I was fortunate to have parents who demonstrated what unconditional love looks like when one of my siblings came out as gay and was accepted with open arms, especially so because of the ongoing AIDS crisis at the time. It taught me that, no matter what, this is and will always be the same child I love and raised. Nothing will ever change that. Do the work to understand what your child is going through, and adapt accordingly. They need you.

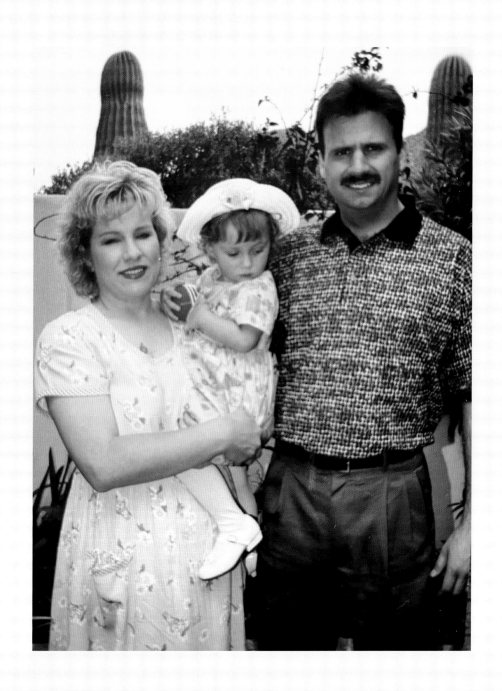

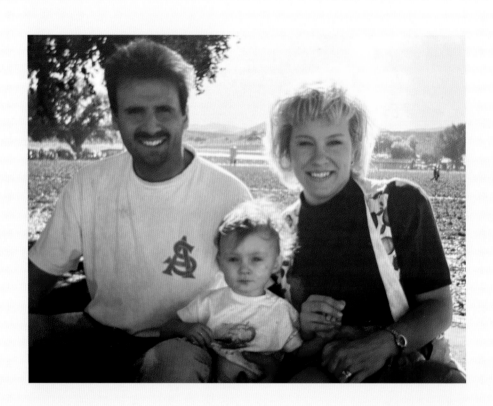

Love Your Child

by Amy Gottlieb

First and foremost, love your child unconditionally. This is not a "choice" for them; it is who they are. It wasn't easy for them to talk with you about something so crucial and personal. You may not understand yet, and you may not be comfortable with what they are telling you, but you need to listen, listen, and listen some more. Ask questions, do your own research, and communicate openly. Love them. Be their safe haven. Be their home.

I had to realize that my dreams for Kade did not match his own. The most important thing is for him to be happy, healthy, and true to himself in every way.

> "Love them. Be their safe haven. Be their home."

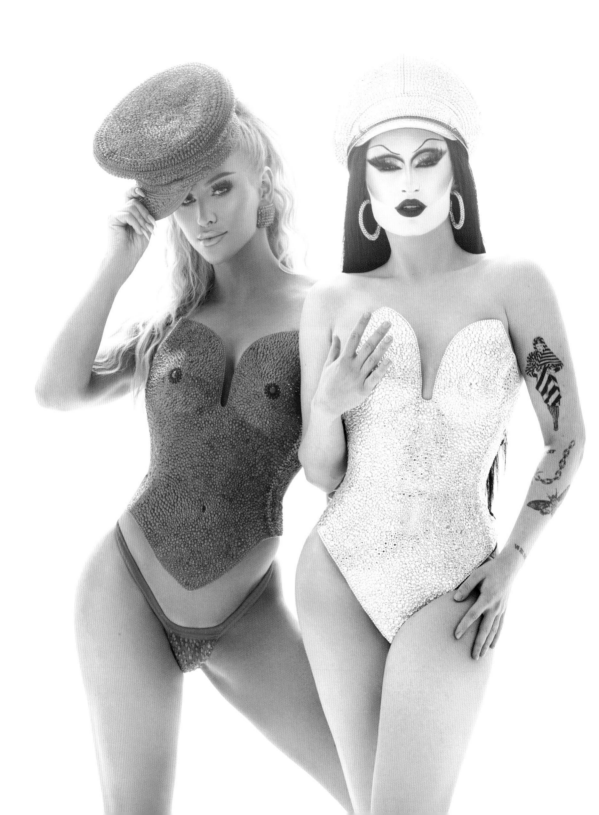

Advice for Cisgender Allies

Cisgender friends, we know you want to be the most amazing allies to the trans people in your life! We also know that how to be a good ally is not self-explanatory. So, we're going to give you a few general pointers. Of course, the best advice is going to come from your trans friend. This is not a one-size-fits-all deal. Everyone has specific preferences when it comes to allyship.

GOTTMIK: My friend Violet Chachki is fearless and selfless when it comes to supporting me. She's basically my bodyguard. Before I got my new ID, my old one made it hard to get into clubs. I was 16 years old in my picture and had long blond hair. The doorman would be like, "Nope," and one second later, Violet would have my Wikipedia page up, ready to fight. Gigi, I think you're the exact same way.

GIGI: Your fight is my fight.

GOTTMIK: Yes. We're all in this together.

GIGI: And everybody has a different journey. The best advice I can give is to be the ally that your friend needs. Just listen. And be willing to show up and fight. That's literally what *ally* means. It's a promise to fight alongside you. If you mess up on pronouns, or you say the wrong name, it's okay. Just correct yourself. Not everybody is as assertive and loud as Violet, which is totally fine. You can quietly show up for your friend. Imagine being a newly trans girl and scared to go out because you're worried somebody's going to call you "he." It's so freeing to have somebody beside you who's going to correct that for you and say, "Actually, it's 'she.'" Another term for getting misgendered is "getting clocked," and it sucks, especially in the beginning. I think the first thing to do as an ally is to get informed about terms like that, and about the rest of the trans landscape.

GOTTMIK: When I was getting misgendered in the beginning, Gigi, you would work in the correct pronoun so casually and gracefully. You'd be like, "Oh, I'll have a Diet Coke, and he will, too."

GIGI: Yeah. Pro tip: don't confront. Just naturally drop the correct pronoun into the conversation.

GOTTMIK: Right. Don't be like, "Actually, he's a boy." Because then the other person feels like they've been shamed.

GIGI: And there's no reason to get defensive. Usually, the other person isn't being malicious. They just don't get it. When you see a newborn baby and assume it's a girl even though it's a boy, the parent doesn't care. They're just like, "Oh, it's a boy." It's not a big deal.

GOTTMIK: Right. If you're an ally, there's a way to stand up for your friend that's noncombative. The correction doesn't have to be a big deal.

GIGI: Another pro tip is to introduce your friend before the other person even has a chance to misgender them.

GOTTMIK: When people used to misgender me and then apologize for it, I'd be like, "Oh, it's fine, it's fine." But saying it was fine was a lie. It wasn't actually fine with me. Another pro tip: don't say it's fine when it's not. Now, I just say, "Thank you," and move on.

GIGI: You gotta keep it moving. And allies have the power to help you do that.

GOTTMIK: The other advice I would give allies is: only be as open as your trans friend wants you to be. If they're not posting about trans pride, for example, then maybe you don't need to. I think a lot of people get confused and think the way to be supportive is to be really loud, but that's not always the case. For example, if an ally mentions their trans friend in a post about trans pride, that could be bad if their mom follows the ally and the trans friend isn't out to their family yet. As an ally, I think the best thing to do is to ask your trans friend how loud they want you to be. Don't make assumptions.

GIGI: Another thing not to do is act like your trans friend isn't actually trans. Once, this friend of mine mentioned her period and then, conspiratorially, said to me, "Oh, us girls."

GOTTMIK: That's just confusing.

GIGI: It made me feel less than. And it gave me the impression that either (a) my friend doesn't think of me as a real woman or (b) she was trying to teach me something about female anatomy. Don't do this, allies. In general, just be really sensitive. Trans people are especially prone to hearing missteps. We have Doberman ears.

GOTTMIK: Another thing not to do is overuse pronouns. No need to be like, "You're just one of the boys today, babe!" If I hear that, then I take it to mean that whoever said it is thinking extra hard about how I'm trans and overcompensating by accentuating the opposite.

GIGI: I have friends who do that. I'll be getting lunch with two girls and they'll be screaming, "Girls day!"

GOTTMIK: No.

GIGI: Yes. And I'm like, "Would you be screaming that if I wasn't here? I don't think so."

GOTTMIK: Right. Get into it, allies, but don't overdo it.

Gottmik's
Hate Crime Experience

I want to share this story as a reminder that, once you do come out and take up space in the world as your authentic self, you have to be prepared for the negatives just as much as you do the positives.

One time, I was doing a Pride event in a small town in middle America. In order to get into the gay club where the event was happening, you had to take an escalator. As I took it up with my friend, a guy was coming down on the other side, and when we passed each other, he reached over the center divide, pushed me, and screamed, "We do not want any transsexuals here!"

I'd always imagined that if someone assaulted me in this way, I'd square up and get super masculine, but in the moment, I was too surprised to react. I had also assumed that if I did ever get assaulted, it would definitely be by someone who was outside the LGBTQIA+ community, not by someone who was supposed to be my ally. My friend ended up chasing the guy away, and I was left feeling shocked and horrified about the hate that had just come at me out of nowhere.

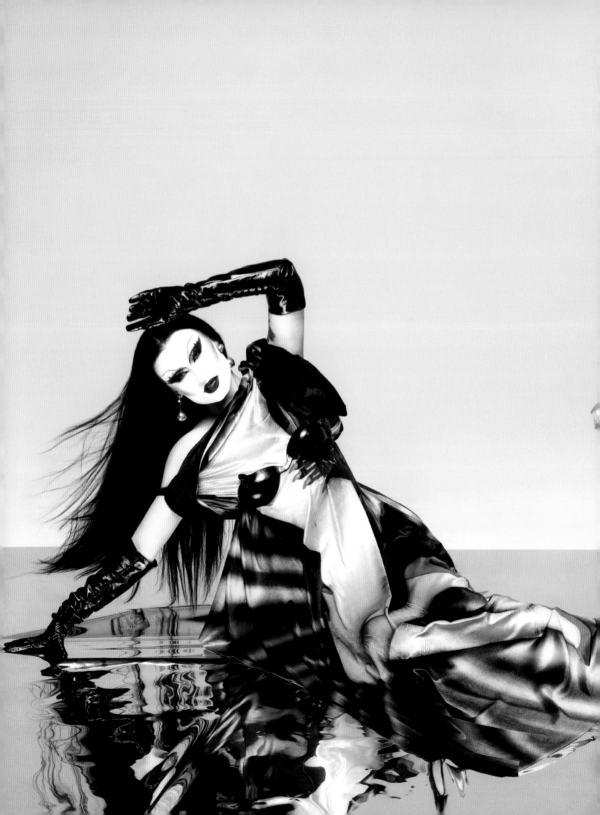

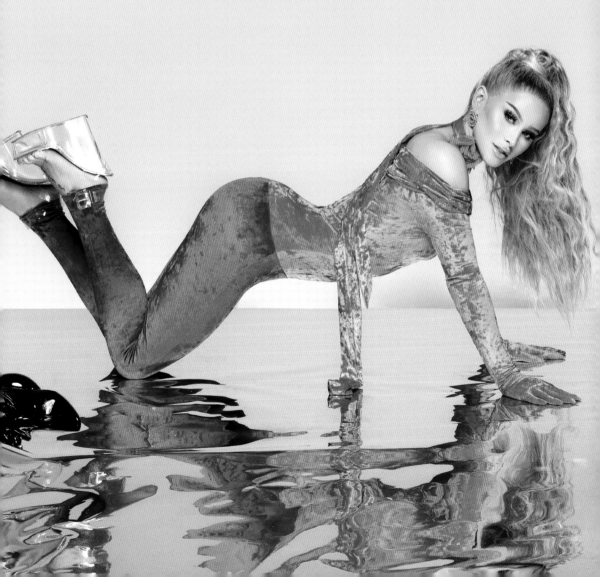

PART 2
TRANSFORMATION

Take Your Time

with **Nats Getty**

PHOTO BY **GIGI GORGEOUS GETTY**

As a kid, strangers often mistook me for a boy. This followed me into adulthood. For years, I was anorexic and addicted to drugs so I had no breasts, which probably helped the confusion. People regularly called me "dude" or "sir." For many, many years, I didn't think much of it—and then I met Gigi and Kade. Watching them transition opened my eyes up to what was possible. It was inspiring to see them embody themselves—to be on the outside who they were on the inside.

During Covid, I had a lot of time to think about my options. Eventually, I decided that I wasn't interested in taking hormones. To be honest, the effects of testosterone on my genitalia was unappealing to me. As somebody who has struggled with body image issues, I didn't think adding a one-inch clit to my life was going to put me in a healthier place. I was also very aware of the pressure I was under. Many trans guys do take hormones, and society's general opinion is that facial hair and a deeper voice equates to masculinity. But did I need to

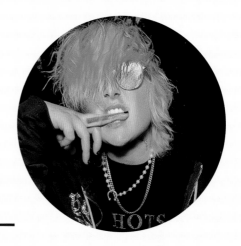

conform to other peoples' ideas about what a man is? No.

What I was absolutely positive about was that I wanted top surgery. My breasts had never felt right to me, and I was sure that after I got them removed, my outsides would match my insides more correctly, and I would feel closer to who I really am. And that was exactly what happened. Now, post-surgery, I am more comfortable with my body. I am more myself.

If anybody is thinking about transitioning, but doesn't want to take hormones, or is on the fence about any other medical augmentation, my advice is to ask yourself, "What do you feel like you need to change?" If you're honest in your answer to that question, you're going to be on a journey that is organic to your needs. I would also suggest starting with the actions that are not irreversible. So, try out a pronoun change, for example, or buy yourself some binders. The transitioning process is long, and there are many steps involved. There is no rush. It's a good idea to take your time.

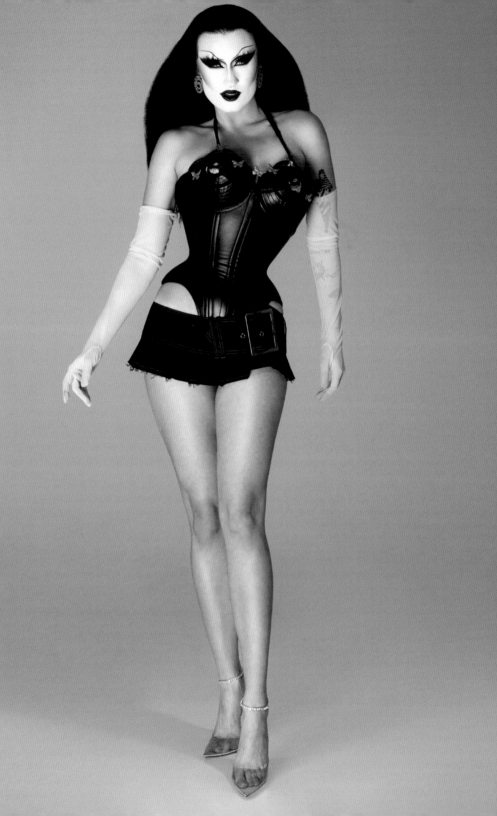

Medical vs. Nonmedical Options

When it comes to the physical aspects of the transitioning process, it's a spectrum. You can get every surgery imaginable, or you can skip all of them. Remember that there is absolutely no rush to decide what you want your transition to look like. Making huge life decisions in a rush is a terrible idea! All ways of transitioning, medical and not, are totally valid. You might feel the pressure to design your journey like somebody else's journey. Don't do that. Keep checking in with yourself. The goal is not to do what other people are doing. It's to do what's in your heart.

GIGI: My transition has been very medical. Taking hormones and doing all the procedures to make me more feminine—I was signing up for all of it from the very beginning. I wanted to be bound to being a female. I never even considered not taking the medical route. From the second I started, I was on a mission to transform my body into the body of a woman with medical help.

GOTTMIK: Same. After I realized I was trans, I felt like I'd spent so much time as a girl against my will. Like I said before, I'm a person who likes to think long and hard about things before announcing them. I did that with hormones. I made an appointment with the LGBT center and told no one. I had to wait about six months for them to see me, which gave me plenty of time to meditate on what I was about to do. During that time, I basically interviewed people from all different points on the spectrum about their experiences, which was super helpful. During those six months, I realized my physical self was a HUGE part of my dysphoria and was really affecting me mentally, and I wouldn't be able to show up 100 percent as myself until I took steps to change my physical appearance

GIGI: Yeah. I really, really wanted hormones in my life, and I still do, because it just makes me feel good. I would say that if it makes you feel good, do it, and if it doesn't make you feel good, then don't do it. That might sound obvious, but there is some pressure in the trans community to take the medical route, so I think it's worth highlighting. It's your transition. Make it work for you. You don't have to take hormones in order for your transition to be valid. A nonmedical transition is just as real as a medical one. It comes down to what you prefer. If you want to try hormones, which is usually the first step, then go for it, but there's no shame if you don't.

GOTTMIK: Yes. I have a lot of followers now who discovered they were trans after seeing me on *Drag Race*. They were like, "Oh, I've always kind of felt like a guy, but I didn't think I could transition because I also have this feminine side." Sometimes I click on their pages and see "he/they" in their bios and look at how amazingly happy they are not medically transitioning, which I love! I think it's so beautiful to be able to know who you are and be comfortable with yourself and those around you to live authentically no matter what! Confidence is key!

GIGI: Yeah, when I transitioned 10 years ago, it didn't even feel like not getting surgery was an option. I remember after I started hormones, everyone was asking me questions like, "When are you getting your boobs done? What about bottom surgery? What about FFS?" [FFS is facial feminization surgery.] Since I looked like a male, it seemed obvious to everyone that I should change parts of my appearance so that I looked more like a female. That was also what I wanted to do, so my feelings were in sync with the popular way to transition at that time. Now, it's no longer like that. Everything is more fluid.

But that doesn't mean the pressure no longer exists. In the trans female community, there are many people who believe that the goal is to be the softest, most beautiful girl—and the most effective way you're going to get there is with hormones and surgery. In the pageant world especially, there's pressure. Actually, a lot of the girls who were competing for the title of Miss Continental, which is an annual female impersonation pageant, transitioned only because they wanted to win.

GOTTMIK: Right. There's a category called "realness." Basically, you go up to the judges and let them touch your skin so they can feel how feminine and smooth it feels.

GIGI: They're checking for stubble. I think some people get addicted to making changes just so they can potentially win. Like, "How much money could I get? Could I be number one?" Adding money and prizes to the equation equals even more pressure. I think the goal is to keep checking in with yourself and asking, *Does this make me happy, or am I overdoing it?* Because plastic surgery can be a slippery slope. Once you start, you want to keep going. Or at least I did.

GOTTMIK: What's interesting is that even though things are much more fluid now, most people still feel the pressure to transition medically.

GIGI: Because in everyday life, while you're out doing your errands or whatever, you want to be recognized as your gender. And I feel like people think that medically transitioning is the best way to make that happen. For me personally, I take it as a compliment when a stranger in a store thinks I'm a girl. It's like, *Yes! I don't have to get misgendered today!*

GOTTMIK: A hundred percent. I'm so comfortable with who I am and love it. But still, to this day, if I'm at a bar and people naturally assume I'm a guy, I feel this instant relief.

GIGI: Yes.

GOTTMIK: It's just the best feeling. For me, when I get these types of comments, it's almost like unnecessary validation for the work I've put into my body and my transition.

GIGI: Mm-hmm. One compliment I always give to trans girls who I think are really pretty is, "Oh my God, I didn't even know," because I know how good it feels when people say that to me. It's just nice to hear, in my opinion, between one trans person and another. But everyone is different. This is not something we recommend cis allies say to a trans person.

GOTTMIK: Right. Even if you're a hundred percent secure in yourself and don't need validation, it's still nice to get the compliment.

GIGI: Another thing about medical procedures is that there are tons of them! So this is not a black-or-white thing. It's more like a road and you choose how far you're going to walk down it. You can just do hormones, or just do hormones and top surgery, etc.

GOTTMIK: Exactly, and I feel like we're going to say this over and over, but you have to keep checking in with yourself. It's okay if you take a lot of time to make these decisions, because they are major.

GIGI: Yeah. Looking back, I wish I had enjoyed every step of my transitioning journey a little more. I was just in such a rush to get everything done. It felt like the clock was ticking … even though it wasn't. I could have gone a lot slower and cherished the moments. I was going so fast that now, I don't even remember when I got my boobs done the first time. Or the second time. I've had them done three times now.

GOTTMIK: Another major thing, if you go the medical route, is choosing the right doctors.

GIGI: So major.

GOTTMIK: Yeah. Looking for doctors is hard, because you want to make sure you vibe with them. You don't want someone who makes you uncomfortable. There's a specific fetishization of the trans community, and sometimes doctors are the ones with the fetish.

GIGI: Absolutely. It's a weird form of power.

GOTTMIK: And sometimes they're so proud that they've found their niche in the trans community. They're like, "I'm a trans doctor, and you need this surgery and that one and this other one." They feel like it's okay to give unsolicited advice. And it's like, *Who asked you?*

GIGI: God complex.

GOTTMIK: Yes. Whoever you choose, you need to meet them in person. Online, they might be the best, but in person they could be the opposite.

GIGI: We're going to tell you who our favorite surgeons are at the end of the book! Flip back there now if you can't wait to find out.

GOTTMIK: And another thing you might consider doing is looking at before-and-after pictures online. I could literally scroll through those all day long. Sometimes when I can't sleep I type "Bottom surgery before and after" into the search bar and scroll through pics for an hour.

GIGI: I mean, yeah, everyone who's considering a medical procedure should be checking out the befores and afters.

GOTTMIK: And doing as much research as possible in general.

GIGI: Yes. The first step is figuring out what you want for yourself, and the next step is getting well informed.

Live Your Own Way

with **Alok**

PHOTO BY **KOHL MURDOCK**

I often say that I wasn't born in the wrong body; I was born in the wrong world. In my experience, I never felt the need for medical procedures to affirm my gender. The dysphoria I experience is not because I personally feel uncomfortable with my body, but because other people misread and misgender me. Gender norms weren't made with me in mind. In fact, in most cases they were made to position communities of color as less-than. My body is nonbinary because I am. The clothes that I wear and the way that I adorn myself are outside of gender because I am.

Transitioning for me was about making the conscious decision to move away from the box "boy" that I was assigned at birth to sharing my nonbinary truth with myself and with the world. It wasn't just about changing the way I presented externally; it was an internal process of self-acceptance, self-declaration, and decolonization. It was about choosing me in a world that makes me have to contour myself into someone else's fiction. It was about acknowledging that I was a soul first, and a body second. It was about sharing my true self with the people I love and being accepted by them for who I am, not for who I should be.

Trans people have always been here and are here to stay. There is no one way to transition, and there are no boxes to be checked off—there is just your way to transition. With the invention of Western colonial medicine people have come to conflate "transition" with "medical transition" and gender exclusively with what we look like, not who we are at a deeper level. Centuries of non-Western and Indigenous understandings and practices around gender and transition were forcibly erased. Nevertheless, trans, Two Spirit, and gender nonconforming communities across the world continue these ways of being and becoming today. Medical gatekeeping doesn't get to dictate the way we live our lives. All transitions and all genders are valid because people own their own bodies and lives.

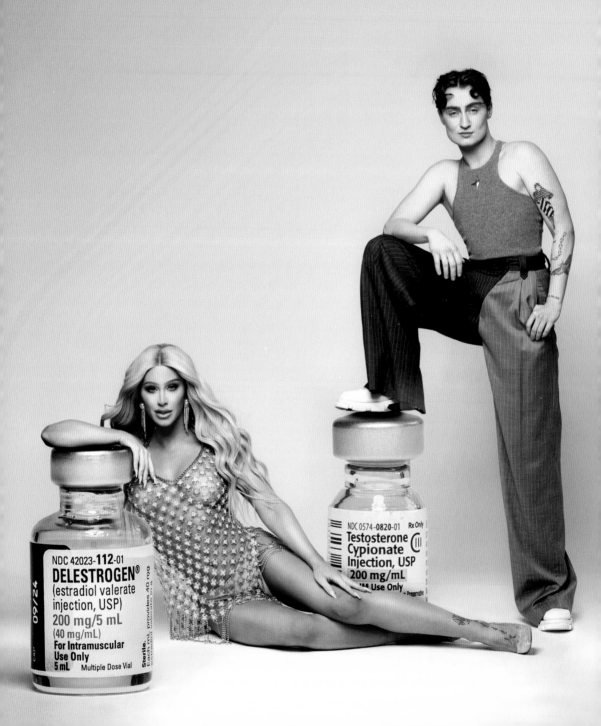

DELESTROGEN®
(estradiol valerate injection, USP)
200 mg/5 mL
(40 mg/mL)
For Intramuscular Use Only
5 mL   Multiple Dose Vial
NDC 42023-**112**-01
EXP 09/24

Testosterone Cypionate Injection, USP
200 mg/mL
IM Use Only   - Preservative
NDC 0574-0820-01   Rx Only

Categories of Medical Transition

In this section, we're going to be covering hormones, top surgery, FFS (facial feminization surgery), bottom surgery, and other, more minimal procedures. We are not doctors. We are just two friends talking about our experiences.

Note

If you're not interested in the elements of a medical transition, then more power to you! Feel free to skip the next section, and we'll pick you up afterward.

Medically Transitioning

PHOTO BY **CORINNE CUMMINGS**

Hi, my name's Jamie and I'm a trans guy from the UK. I'm 28, been on testosterone for over a decade, had top and bottom surgery, and I'm really comfortable and proud with who I am.

I had metoidioplasty (or meta) when I was 23, about six years after I started hormones. I say this because some people think transitioning is really quick, but that's not the case! I was pretty quick to realize I was trans when I heard the term watching TV at 16. I was also pretty quick to know that I needed hormones and top surgery to relieve a lot of my gender dysphoria. But when it came to

bottom surgery, it took me a little longer to know if this was something I needed to do enough to go through surgery again, and then deciding which type of surgery was best for me. There's no such thing as "the surgery," just like there's no one way to be trans, so I took my time to figure it out.

I mostly did this by watching YouTube videos of people talking about their experiences. (The irony being that as a creator, I now do this on my own channel!) I also did my own research online, including looking at sites where people anonymously posted their results. In

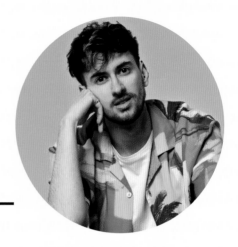

the end, I decided meta was the best option for me. It was personally important to minimize my scarring, and while phallo [phalloplasty] leads to … larger results, size wasn't important to me. (Feel free to research these on your own time.) I was nervous to have another surgery. It's never a nice thing to do and I knew the recovery would be longer than top surgery, but it felt right, and like the beginning of the final step I needed to kick my dysphoria's butt!

Waking up post-op, I had a HUGE sense of relief that it had been done, but wow were things tender! I ended up having some recovery complications, too, but after a week, I was recovering at home, and a few days later I could hobble up and down the stairs. The catheter finally came out after two weeks, and from there it was pretty smooth sailing. Despite the complications, this surgery is something I'm super grateful to have gotten done. It's improved the way I feel about myself and reduced my dysphoria more than I ever thought it would. Not everybody knows straightaway, and surgery is a big deal, so it's okay to be nervous. Take your time, and ultimately do whatever is best for you!

Category is: Hormones (aka 'Mones)

Hormones are usually the first step on the medical transition journey. Trans girls take estrogen, trans guys take testosterone, and nonbinary people might take either. This is not a one-stop shop. If you like what the hormones are doing for you, you'll keep taking them—for as long as you want, and maybe forever. Side effects for trans girls generally include softer, smoother skin, and trans guys get the opposite: rougher skin and increased hair and bottom growth. The biggest difference, though, is voice. Testosterone lowers your voice, and estrogen doesn't affect your voice at all.

GOTTMIK: As I mentioned earlier, I booked an appointment to get hormones at the LGBT center and then kept it a secret for six months. On the day I went to get my first injection of testosterone, I FaceTimed you, Gigi, and Nats and I was like, "I'm doing this. I didn't tell you guys. I'm so scared." I had the worst needle fear ever. I don't have that so much anymore, but back then I did. You and Nats were the best people to call. You totally understood and said all the right things. Then, the second the testosterone got injected, and it was game over. It just felt so right. I had never felt that in my life. I was like, *Excuse me? Did my depression just get cured?* That, to me, was proof that I was doing exactly what I was meant to be doing.

GIGI: A hundred percent. When I got my first shot and took my pills for the first time, a huge weight was lifted. After I met my mentor, Betty, and her circle of trans women, it became very clear to me that I wanted to take the medical route. They showed me what the end goal was. When I met them, I was shocked by how beautiful they were and how happy they seemed. At the time, people were often confused by my gender. I was a boy wearing girl's clothes and people would ask me constantly if I was a girl or a boy. Before I found Betty and her friends, I was saying, "Oh, I'm a boy. Don't even worry about it."

I wasn't fully aware of how much I had needed hormones until I started taking them. I didn't know that feeling so much better in my body was even an option. I loved the physical effects, and I loved the emotional effects, too. As a kid, I'd had such a problem with empathy. I never cried. I wasn't very good at putting myself in somebody else's shoes.

Well, after about a month on hormones, I had all kinds of feelings I didn't even know I could have. It was strange at first, and also really interesting. It allowed me to start seeing myself in a new way. Eventually, after a few more months, my emotions evened out, and I just got more used to them.

What I would say to anyone who's about to embark on the hormone journey is to really take time to feel out the side effects, because it can be jarring at first. I personally know a bunch of people who've tried hormones and didn't love them. So, they stopped. That's what's great about hormones—you can always slow the process down a bit. Just make sure you do your research because there are some irreversible side effects.

GOTTMIK: My skin started producing oils I had never had before, and I broke out in the craziest acne! The very first thing I noticed, though, before any physical or emotional side effects, was that my voice dropped.

GIGI: Voice is a thing.

GOTTMIK: It's such a thing—for trans guys. Even though all side effects vary from person to person, most people get a deeper voice after they start taking testosterone.

GIGI: Estrogen, on the other hand, doesn't change your voice at all. Once you've gone through puberty, your voice drops and just stays down there. And yes, as you said, with testosterone, the effects are dramatic.

GOTTMIK: Testosterone basically puts you through male puberty and pretty much everything changes: your voice, your orgasms, your body, where your fat distributes. Everything is just completely different, whereas estrogen doesn't do most of that. You just get really pretty skin.

GIGI: And different fat distribution.

GOTTMIK: Right. You get boobs.

GIGI: Tiny ones, at least for me. They're more like fat pockets. But some people have larger ones, too. Most people I know have gotten implants.

GOTTMIK: Right. A lot of elements of transitioning have layers in that way. You can choose to just do the estrogen and enjoy your natural boobs, or you can go a step further and get the implants. It's the same with voice. You can just take testosterone, or you can take it and train your voice to be lower, for example. I didn't end up training my voice because the change was so dramatic. Everybody commented on it.

GIGI: Yeah. When we watch old videos of you, it's startling how high your voice is!

GOTTMIK: Seriously, and it happened fast, too. By the end of one month on testosterone, my voice had changed a little, and by month three, it was very noticeable. It's kind of hard to assess the changes for yourself, since it's happening little by little every day. It didn't actually hit me how much my voice had changed until I watched one of those old videos of myself. I could not believe how high-pitched I sounded. It surprised me a lot, because it's not like I'd gone out of my way to make my voice more masculine. I was just speaking naturally, not trying at all. Honestly, when I saw the old video and compared it to my new voice, it was the best thing in the world. It just confirmed even more that I was on the right path. I mean, I'm not a huge fan of the balding, but other than that, all the changes have been stunning.

GIGI: Balding is brutal.

GOTTMIK: My hairline used to be round. And now I literally have this widow's peak. Which is common. Just your basic male pattern baldness.

GIGI: I was so insecure about my voice back in the day. I used to have this tiny hack on YouTube to make me sound more feminine. First, I would shoot my whole video. And then once I was done editing it, I would speed it up to 103 or 104 beats per minute, because doing that pitched my voice up a little bit. I remember my manager, Scott, texted me while I was shooting one of the videos, and the sound of the phone was so insanely high-pitched, to a cartoon-like level, not believable at all. Later, Scott was like, "Did you speed up your video? The text alert on your phone sounds crazy. And you're talking really fast." And I was like, "No! What? It must be a YouTube glitch!" But people in the comments would call me out, too. And I was just so insecure about it that I blamed YouTube every time.

The best advice that I can give about this is that you just have to find a pitch that's right for you. I hear a lot of trans girls overdoing it. And I understand why they feel compelled to do that. The voice thing can be such a source of insecurity.

GOTTMIK: Yeah, I feel like if someone is questioning your gender, they're waiting to hear your voice so they can figure it out.

GIGI: Yes. A doctor told me once that within three to five seconds of seeing your face, people decide if you're a boy or a girl. You can change the features of your face with surgery and other procedures, but trans girls can't change their voice in a major way. The register is just lower than a cis woman's. People hear it and immediately think, *Oh, this is a man.*

When I was first transitioning, I was staying in a lot of hotels, and I remember calling room service to see if I would get a "sir" or a "ma'am." I was trying to figure out how to make my new voice sound cute—without overdoing it. Oh my God, thinking back on this makes me realize how uncomfortable the voice thing used to make me. Now I feel much more relaxed about it.

GOTTMIK: I'm very thankful my voice dropped; it's definitely eased a bit of my dysphoria. And you can get surgery on your vocal cords, but it's risky.

GIGI: So risky. When I got my trachea shaved, the doctor said we could do my vocal cords, too. Even back in the day, when I was shameless and in a mad rush to get everything done, I was like, "No."

GOTTMIK: We know people whose voices never came back after that surgery.

GIGI: It's so scary.

GOTTMIK: You literally lose your voice forever.

GIGI: It's horrifying. I mean, vocal cords are so fragile.

GOTTMIK: I know for a fact I would a hundred percent do it. Because if I still had my old voice, I wouldn't be able to live. When I call room service and get a "ma'am," I'm like, *Oh my God no.*

GIGI: When I first started transitioning, I was in an Uber in New York City with my friend/mentor Betty. It was late at night and we'd been out partying so my guard was down. I said to the driver, "Sir, can you turn up the music?" And he was like, "Okay, sir, no problem."

GOTTMIK: No.

GIGI: Yes. I feel it's so important, especially for trans girls, to find a pitch that is natural and sustainable. Definitely don't murder yourself over it. For me, one of the reasons I stopped trying so hard to change my voice was because I realized it's my job. People would hear me speak and be like, "Oh, I recognize you by your voice." It was better if I sounded just like, well, myself.

GOTTMIK: I get so triggered when I think I sound too feminine, but the other thing is that it's hard to hear yourself (and see yourself) clearly. We are focusing on the imperfections, but other people probably aren't.

GIGI: Right, so true.

GOTTMIK: Training your voice to change with voice therapy isn't the worst option, because it's noninvasive.

GIGI: Yeah, I know a couple of people who've done that on YouTube. You basically listen to a sentence and then repeat it in a higher pitch.

GOTTMIK: There are also these vibrational meditations you can find online that allegedly alter your vocal chords. I've turned one of those on and put my phone on my chest in the hopes that the vibrations would lower my voice while I was sleeping.

GIGI: Did it work?

GOTTMIK: I have no idea. I've only done it a few times. Maybe I should get back into it, though, because if I could have a deeper voice, then sign me up.

GIGI: Yeah. I mean, I feel like I've organically trained my voice over time and now, when I speak, it just comes out at a certain pitch. I can't even remember what my voice sounded like before transitioning. I do have to say, though, that when I walk into a room full of strangers, I turn the voice up a notch. I'm like, "Hey, honey!" I feel like a lot of trans girls do that.

GOTTMIK: Sure, and I think a lot of trans guys, especially ones who want to present as super masculine, lower the pitch in a room full of strangers.

GIGI: If you're wondering how to deal with this, I say keep testing it out until you find a pitch that works for you. And if you want to get a sense of how people will read you, then call a random number and say, "Hi."

GOTTMIK: I want to quickly mention another change that not many people talk about: bottom growth on testosterone. Basically, your clitoris grows up to 3 inches in size. There wasn't a crazy amount of information about this when I started, so it kind of freaked me out at first, but let me tell you, it really does! It really does look and function like a small penis. I can get hard and everything! I went from being scared of it happening to wanting more. I definitely want to take the next step in my medical transition and do a surgery called metoidioplasty, where they basically elongate your t-dick a bit more and pull your urethra out of it so you can pee standing up. Now that would truly be a game changer for me!

Category is: Top Surgery, FFS, Etc.

For many transgender people, the next phase of medically transitioning includes top surgery. Some trans girls get breast implants. Trans guys often get a subcutaneous mastectomy. Trans girls are generally left with a smaller, less visible scar, while the scar after top surgery for guys (depending on the type of surgery) is generally larger. If you're interested in minimizing its appearance, this can be just as important as the surgery itself.

Another option for trans girls at this point in the transition is FFS, or facial feminization surgery. This single term can encompass a broad number of procedures that are designed to give the face a more feminine appearance. For many trans girls, this is important, because the face is what people see first. The list of procedures under the FFS umbrella might include forehead contouring, eye and eyelid modification, cheek augmentation, nose reshaping, lip lift, jaw angle reduction, chin width reduction, tracheal shave, lowering the hairline, and hair transplantation.

GOTTMIK: I think I started researching top surgery the instant I realized that I might be trans. I had never considered it before that in any serious way, which is weird, because I had never liked my breasts. They just felt so wrong to me, like they didn't belong on my body.

About a year into my transition, on Thanksgiving, you, Gigi, and Nats told me you were going to pay for it, because I didn't have a lot of money at the time. It was the best day of my life, and the best gift I have ever received.

GIGI: Aw, we're so cute.

GOTTMIK: So cute.

GIGI: After I got my top surgery, I looked at myself in the mirror and I didn't cry or scream or anything. I wasn't that emotional, because I didn't feel that surprised. I just thought, *Oh, my body finally matches what my brain has been seeing for a long time.* It felt like I was finally putting the pieces together. It was just so right.

GOTTMIK: Same. Getting the 'mones was the first major sign that I was on the right path, and top surgery was second. It was just like, *Yes!*

GIGI: Yes. I've had my boobs done three times now. I think the most recent one was the best.

GOTTMIK: You look fabulous.

GIGI: As do you. You've done such a good job of taking care of your scars. You need to talk about that. I feel that for guys, the scars are as important as the surgery.

GOTTMIK: Oh, yes. This process has actually turned me into a connoisseur of scar remedies. What I did was research everything to death. From my research, I kind of created my own process. I'm not saying this is going to work for everyone, but it's worked pretty well for me so far.

For the first six months after surgery, I applied the same brand of scar patches that Serena Williams used after her C-section. They're by a company called embrace Active Scar Defense, and they're kind of expensive, but they are great at helping to prevent your skin from stretching. One rule after top surgery for some trans guys is that you're not allowed to lift your arms up over your head for six months, by the way, which is really annoying and hard. I definitely struggled with this.

After the six months of wearing the scar patches, I tried laser therapy, which is a popular option. It's basically what the internet tells you to do. The purpose is to get rid of redness and prevent keloids, or raised scars. I personally did not love the effects of laser therapy, so I found a different procedure that had much better results for me. It's called scar camouflaging. It's similar to microneedling. I saw Dr. Basma Hameed in Beverly Hills. Everyone's body is different, and the number of sessions varies. I was told I'd need about four sessions. I've had one so far, and my scars look so much better. You can also inject your scars with a solution that flattens them. Basically, there are a lot of options, and probably everyone's skin is going to be affected in a slightly different way.

GIGI: Absolutely.

"What I did was research everything to death. From my research, I kind of created my own process."

GOTTMIK: Okay, now you need to talk about FFS.

GIGI: A big one. Basically, facial feminization surgery transforms masculine features from the neck up into feminine features. Before FFS, I had never really realized which parts of my face made people read me as male. I was like, *What does my forehead have to do with it?* Well, it turns out there are tons of differences between cisgender men and cisgender women when it comes to the face. Men tend to have a ridge above their eyes called a "caveman brow," for example, whereas on women, that area is generally flat.

I remember after I recovered, I did my makeup, and I couldn't believe how much bigger and prettier my eyes looked without that ridge. Strangers called me "she" and "her" so much more often. It was a big thing that I didn't expect to be so major.

GOTTMIK: And all of those procedures are done at once, right?

GIGI: Yeah. And I recommend it. I mean, I'm pro surgery. I think if you want it done and you can afford it, then why not? But, as I said before, just know that it can be a slippery slope. Once you get one thing done, you might just get fixated on something else.

GOTTMIK: What I did was I basically took FFS and I flipped it to create my own version of FMS. I guess we could call it facial masculinization surgery. Technically, it doesn't exist, but it should.

Basically, I took all the elements of a masculine face and tried to emulate them using various methods. I wanted to square out my face as much as possible, so I literally created a new jaw and chin with filler. I've noticed that when I have bigger eyebrows, it kind of takes away from the lack of not having a brow bone, so I made my eyebrows extra bushy by tattooing "hair" around them. Usually, it is more stereotypically masculine to have lower eyebrows and more stereotypically feminine to have more space between the eyelids and the eyebrows. So in photos I'm always kind of pushing my eyebrows down. I've learned that Botox lowers them a little bit, too. Taking T [testosterone] isn't necessarily supposed to give you an Adam's apple, but I think it definitely did just a little for me. Sometimes, I'll even contour it a bit with makeup.

GIGI: There's a lot you can do if you understand the masculine and feminine features of the face.

GOTTMIK: And I would say that if you're uncomfortable with one of your features, don't be afraid to change it, and don't be afraid to trust your intuition. I invented a lot of the things that I did, just because it seemed intuitive to me. I've had doctors say, "I never even thought of that!" Well, none of my doctors have been trans, so why would they have thought of it?

GIGI: I have a story about this. A while back, a woman who was doing my hair asked me how I got my lips so high. She was like, *I want that. Is it filler?* I told her that no, I got plastic surgery. She went to her doctor, who laughed and said that lip lifts are just for old people!

GOTTMIK: Right. So, at the end of the day, nobody else knows what you need. You know what you need.

GIGI: Exactly.

Category is: Bottom Surgery

Bottom surgery is usually last on the list, because it's such a big deal. For both trans guys and girls, this procedure is complex and irreversible. Neither of us has had bottom surgery yet, but we both want it, so in this conversation, we are weighing the pros and cons and going through our options. We are not speaking from direct experience.

GOTTMIK: For me, transitioning has been a very emotional and spiritual journey so far. A lot of what has shifted is internal, but the external has an effect on the internal, of course. As a trans person, I struggle to feel connected to my body. Every day, I'm making an effort to love my body and feel comfortable in it. I want to look in the mirror and say, "Oh yes, that's me."

When it comes to bottom surgery, part of me wonders why I think I need it. Because it would be just for me and whoever I have sex with. Nobody else would know. So, is it worth it? This is a question I've asked myself so many times. What I've come to realize is that in order for me to love myself in the way I want to love myself, and in order for me to love somebody else in the way that I want to love somebody else, it's going to be worth it. I don't think I necessarily *need* bottom surgery, but I do think I would love it.

A huge consideration is where we are medically with this as a society. As with a lot of trans procedures, bottom surgery hasn't been perfected yet. It's still in process, which is kind of scary, especially for trans guys. There are two options, *metoidioplasty* and *phalloplasty*, and neither of them are my perfect dream penis scenario. With phalloplasty, they take out a graft out of your forearm or your leg. It goes pretty deep.

What is the difference between metoidioplasty and phalloplasty?

Metoidioplasty: a gender-affirming, lower body surgery that creates a penis by cutting ligaments around the erectile tissue (clitoris) to release it from the pubis and give the shaft more length!

Phalloplasty: a lower body surgery performed to construct, repair, or enlarge the penis.

Note: While not discussed at length in this chapter, other types of bottom surgery include labiaplasty, orchiectomy, scrotectomy, urethroplasty, vaginoplasty, and vulvaplasty. We encourage additional research, as needed.

GIGI: And the skin never raises again in that area. It stays dropped.

GOTTMIK: Yes, it's definitely a tough surgery.

          They make a penis out of a piece of skin, basically, but it can't get hard on its own. You have to pump it or put something in it to make it erect before sex. There are a couple of different ways to do that, and all of them don't seem ideal to me. Do I want to pause to pump before having sex with my boyfriend? I'm not sure I would love that for me right now.

          Metoidioplasty is another option. Like we were talking about earlier, when you're on testosterone, your t-dick lengthens, and this procedure lengthens it even more so that it grows closer to the size of a cisgender man's dick. And you can get balls implanted, too.

GIGI: And then there's the orgasm component.

GOTTMIK: Right. If the metoidioplasty is successful, then I'd have the same type of orgasms that I have currently. Which, by the way, are so different now that I'm on testosterone. The female orgasm is more of an all-body sensation, and the orgasm on testosterone is much more centralized, and weirdly addictive.

          As of right now, I'm really happy with my growth down there. So, if it were a little longer, I think I'd be even happier. Like I said before, I would love to be able to pee standing up. That would be so amazing. I want to consider the phalloplasty situation, but right now, I'm not sure that I'm comfortable with where we are medically with it. I think the art of the phalloplasty can be perfected a lot more.

GIGI: Some doctors seriously need to figure this out. It's weird that they haven't yet.

GOTTMIK: I know. The vagina surgery, meanwhile, is stunning.

GIGI: It really is. So, backing up for a second, I paid for my face myself, and my boobs, and when my dad finally came around to accepting that I was trans, he called me and said, "I'm going to pay you back for all of those surgeries and I want to pay for your vagina, too." I thought, *Great, I'm doing this, I'm going to find a doctor.*

Then I moved to LA and checked in with myself. I was like, *Do I really need one?* In my mind, I already had one. Going to the bathroom obviously wasn't great, but my dysphoria wasn't crippling either. Meanwhile, my dad, who'd finally gotten on board, would be calling me, asking, "When are we booking the surgery?" He couldn't wrap his head around the fact that I didn't want a vagina ASAP.

Now, I'm in a new place. I've decided I definitely want one. I don't know who the doctor's going to be yet, or when I'm going to do it, but I feel confident that it will be successful. I've always dreamed of wearing women's underwear. I know I'm going to be obsessed. I can't wait to burn all my old underwear. So, for me, getting bottom surgery is not urgent, but when it happens, it's going to feel magical. I will be doing it purely for me, because I want to. It has nothing to do with social pressure.

GOTTMIK: Yeah, I had to really make sure that I wasn't wanting to get bottom surgery because that's what I think society needs from me. I also wonder how society will change in the future. Are we always going to assign gender by sex? I hope not.

Part of my wanting bottom surgery has to do with the way I like to hook up with guys. I sometimes like to top, meaning that if I want to hook up with someone, I have to pause to strap something on. I know this only takes a second to do, but I am so over it. I don't want to do it anymore. The guys I hook up with don't necessarily care. But *I* care. So, I can live—I *am* living—without it, but I think having the surgery would make sex feel more natural.

GIGI: For a lot of girls and guys, this is the last step of their transition. So, I feel that by the time you arrive here, you've done a lot of work changing your body and your mind. Hopefully you feel a lot more peaceful. Your name has probably been changed. So many of the boxes have been checked, and this is the last thing. It's bigger than a nose job, or a brow bone shave, or cheek implants, or whatever else. But unlike those other procedures, it's literally just for you.

GOTTMIK: Right. I wasn't sure that I wanted bottom surgery until I got comfortable with my pansexuality. I hooked up with a lot of guys and a lot of girls and realized that I just wasn't interested in a more submissive role. Coming to terms with how I want to have sex was really the turning point for me in terms of bottom surgery.

GIGI: When do you think you're going to get it, realistically?

GOTTMIK: Soon-ish.

GIGI: Can you do that and then the phalloplasty after?

GOTTMIK: Yeah, you can.

GIGI: It's like a revision. But once you do that, it's over. It's changed, right?

GOTTMIK: Forever.

GIGI: I can handle a lot of surgeries, but bottom surgery makes me anxious.

GOTTMIK: I know. It's such a special area.

GIGI: And then there are the people I know who've second-guessed doing it.

GOTTMIK: You have to be so sure.

GIGI: So, so sure.

Jazz Jennings *on*
The Importance of Gender-Affirming Care

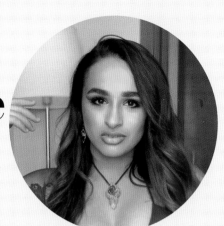

PHOTO BY **JEANETTE JENNINGS**

Receiving gender-affirming care changed my life.

I socially transitioned when I was five, so I was fortunate to be able to go on puberty blockers and cross hormones before developing secondary male characteristics. When I was 17, I underwent gender confirmation surgery to complete my transition from male to female. On the day of my vaginoplasty surgery, I was beyond euphoric because I knew I was about to experience an operation I had anticipated my whole life.

I feel blessed that I was given the opportunity to receive the medical care I needed. To this day, I am so happy with my transition and the steps I took to become the woman I am today. I am proud of my trans identity, and I am proud to be me. Gender-affirming care saved my life, and I'm forever grateful to all the professionals who made my dreams of fully transitioning come true.

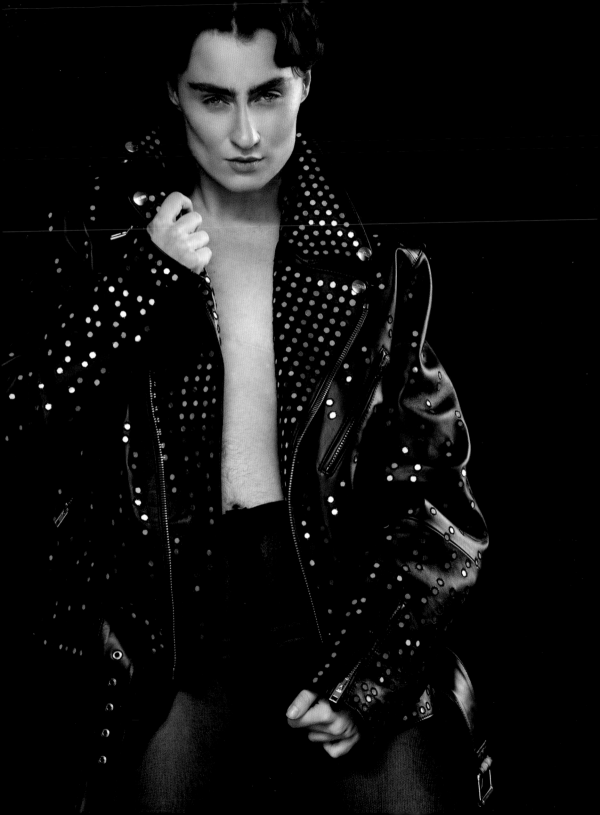

Realistic Expectations

It's best not to assume that just because you've transitioned, the world has transitioned alongside you. The truth is that most people are thinking about themselves most of the time, which means that the comments and weird looks that might come your way really shouldn't be taken that personally. But, you're only human, and some days, you're going to feel triggered by how the world receives you. Just because you're dressing differently and you've changed your voice and you've possibly had some medical procedures done does not mean that you're never going to get clocked again.

The most helpful expectation to have is that your transition is going to take time. It's never going to be fully over, either. It's so important to be patient and loving with yourself during the process, because transitioning is not an easy thing. It takes guts.

GIGI: I actually got my FFS done before I did my boobs, because I didn't want to walk around with big boobs and a manly face. So, the FFS, as I said before, was my first major surgery. And leading up to it, I was like, "I need this. I need this." I couldn't wait to get it. I thought it was going to change my life completely. Like, I basically thought I was going to become the prettiest, softest Victoria's Secret Model–esque girl in the world.

But that's not what happened. After I got the FFS and I was living with my new face, I still experienced the ups and downs that I had experienced before. I was still the same person. Some days, I was easily triggered. Other days, I wasn't.

I think it's really important for people to know that medical procedures are not a be-all, end-all. They don't change your personality. You're still you. Which is why it's crucial that you get your mind in the right place before you start changing the physical stuff. Like you said before, Gottmik, getting in touch with the emotional and spiritual aspects of this journey should come first. If you don't do that, then you might be disappointed.

GOTTMIK: Yeah, medical procedures definitely don't change you as a person.

GIGI: They're a little bonus.

GOTTMIK: Before I got top surgery, I would wear binders. Even when I was out at night, I'd wear half ones. And sometimes someone would hug me and I could feel their hands touch my back right at the edge of the binder, and I would freak out. I'd be like, *Oh my God, they can feel my binder right now. This is the worst thing in the world.* I mean, I went into a total spiral just because somebody touched my back. It was crazy. I'd be like, *I have to go home right this second*. And then I would literally leave.

This tiny detail—or what probably would seem like a tiny detail to a lot of people—was so huge for me. It would ruin my night. Which is all to say that yes, of course you have to get right in your mind before you start changing your body. If you do that, then the bonus of getting some of these procedures can feel incredible. Because they can bring you closer to your conception of yourself as a physical being. If you don't know who you are or what you really want, then how can you get closer to yourself?

GIGI: I think getting your mind right could be defined as developing a sense of comfort with who you are—on a soul level. No matter how many changes you make to your body, you could still get clocked. That's just part of what it means to be trans for most people. After I got my boobs done, I thought I'd be less insecure, but then I just became insecure about something else. Which is very human and okay. It's just about having realistic expectations. After I stopped expecting whatever procedure to make me happier, I felt a huge sense of relief.

GOTTMIK: Right. I could have a full fucking beard and a six pack and be shirtless and someone could still call me "she" for whatever reason. I don't actually know why, but my brain is really good at making up reasons. I'll think, *Oh, it's because of my walk*, or, *Oh, it's because I gained weight and my hips are bigger right now.* There's always going to be something that I'm just going to fixate on. I've accepted that. One super helpful thing to remember is that whoever is doling out the comments is not thinking about you. Everybody's on their own journey.

GIGI: The other thing is that you never get to a finish line. It's not a race with a beginning and an end. It's a process, and it continues to be a process. I haven't had bottom surgery yet, but I assume that after I do, I'm not going to feel done. I'm going to keep working on myself, both inside and out. I'm so happy I'm taking this time to pause right now before bottom surgery. Before, I was just thinking, *After I get everything done, I am going to be happy.* I know this is what a lot of girls think. And it's just not true. You're not going to be plucked out of your unhappiness just because you have boobs. I have a feeling that social media is partially responsible for spreading the illusion that transitioning is easy and everyone who transitions is content. Um, they're not. Trans people are like everybody else. We're all just trying.

"...you have to keep asking yourself, 'What am I believing right now?'"

GOTTMIK: I think most people get to a place where they are comfortable and happy to some degree. Everyone has their own pace and their own idea of what their transition should look like and what it means to them.

GIGI: It just takes time. I think that's a good expectation to have. Expect it to take time.

GOTTMIK: And expect the possibility that you'll never truly be done. We as humans always try to find flaws and think we have to fix everything, which is why finding true self-love and confidence is extremely crucial.

GIGI: Right. How often do people look out the window and say, "Wow, isn't life just so beautiful?" People rarely do that. They're more likely to say something like, "I'm worried I'm going to be late," or "I'm so stressed about this meeting I have later." This is how trans people feel about their gender. Rarely do we say, "Wow, aren't I just so beautiful?"

GOTTMIK: We forget to be grateful.

GIGI: Because we're focused on problems instead. I know a few girls who have had their faces fully done, and they've gotten the most gorgeous boobs ... and they are some of the most insecure, unwell girls I've ever met. It's all in your mind. Whatever you believe ends up being your reality. Which is why you have to keep asking yourself, "What am I believing right now?"

GOTTMIK: Yes.

GIGI: This might sound silly, but maybe every day, create a little plan for yourself in the morning. You could say what you're grateful for and maybe write a journal entry so that you can be tracking your thoughts and your emotional progress as you make your way through your journey. Looking back, I can see that this is what I was doing with my YouTube videos. It was my way of keeping a diary—with an audience.

GOTTMIK: I mean, I feel like I hear people say this all the time: "It's a journey, and you have to take it step by step and make sure you're cherishing every day." It's probably good advice, but I have not listened to it. I've been like, "I do not want to cherish any of these steps. I just want to get through this and get over it and move on to the next thing."

          I see a lot of trans guys online tracking progress with their voice. They'll be like, "This is my voice after one day on testosterone. This is my voice after one month on testosterone." So, it's the same as what you did, Gigi. It's like keeping a journal with an audience.

          My process has been more internal and quieter. I needed the first few months on T to just be with myself so I could figure out what I was thinking. One potential hazard of sharing is that then people have opinions that they want you to know about. I just couldn't handle any of that. Sometimes I wonder how the amount of estrogen in my body played a role. I mean, normally, I like to work things out for myself, but before the T really kicked in, I did feel like I needed to hibernate and be gentle.

GIGI: That's interesting. I wonder if part of the reason I wanted to speed through the process was because my testosterone was higher in the beginning. I just had a blast of new energy, and I was like, "Let's fucking do this!"

GOTTMIK: I think the estrogen in my system might have made me a bit more sentimental at first.

GIGI: That makes sense. I feel we need to touch upon what it's like right after surgery, too. The first day is the hardest. And then you get more and more used to it day after day. You'll definitely have setbacks. We all do. And that will suck. But then maybe you'll have a great day and not get misgendered at all. No matter what, just keep getting yourself out there. You want to be independent and tenacious.

GOTTMIK: It does get easier overall, but you will still have your days. And life will still be life-y. It's not like your problems pause because you're transitioning. A few years into my transition, I broke my arm, and I was left with this giant scar, which sent me into a total meltdown. I was like, *Oh my God, I'm already trans. I'm finally just now changing the parts of my body that I have hated forever. I'm working so hard to get to a place where I feel comfortable in my skin. All I want is to look in the mirror and like what I see.* And then I had to break my arm and have this ginormous scar on my arm against my will? It just seemed like yet another inconvenience for this body that's been inconvenienced for most of its life. And it seemed like a waste of effort on my part. I thought, *What's the point of working so hard at making my body beautiful if I can't even keep it intact?* It truly sent me to a place of hopelessness. I think it's probably safe to say that you should expect to feel frustrated and sad sometimes. That's normal. Maybe some days, you'll find the inner strength to push through. And other days, you might just need to cry. It's all valid!

GIGI: Affirmations might seem cheesy to you, but that could be a great thing to do when you're feeling down. I feel it's important to find an affirmation that works for you. You can target a trait you want, like, "I am worthy," or "I am powerful." Or you can target specific goals. Do you want to be a pro tennis player? Do you want to be the best housewife on Earth? Do you want to be an iconic designer? Whatever it is, say it out loud and say it all the time. I feel the more you repeat your affirmation, the more you'll start to believe it.

GOTTMIK: My version of that pick-me-up is comparing myself now to who I was in middle school or high school. I envision the younger me being thrilled about how things have turned out so far. If you would have told me at in high school, "Everything is going to be okay. You're going to have these amazing friends and this amazing job and you're going to live in LA," I would have felt so relieved. Because back then, I was worried about how things would turn out, and I wasn't sure that I was trans yet, and it was just confusing. This exercise reminds me, too, that in the future, my life is going to be even bigger and better—I hope.

GIGI: On that note, what I can say is that now that I've been transitioning for 10 years, I have a lot of younger versions of myself who would have been so excited to see me now. Back in the day, I was definitely a lot more insecure. And now I just feel at peace with who I am. There is no magic formula for achieving serenity as a trans person. It just takes time. And courage.

I'm proud to say that I really did have courage when I was younger. I lived so fully. I threw myself into LA life and threw myself into relationships. I was fully independent and fearless in a way. I said yes to a lot; I met a lot of people; I had a lot of fun. I didn't have much of a support system to fall back on, except for my chosen family. Now I can see that the trials and tribulations of my youth really shaped who I am.

If you're able to, I strongly suggest that you throw yourself into the world like I did. You'll learn to navigate any situation, and you'll get much better at pulling yourself out of a negative rut, because you'll have more experience. When something hard happens, you'll say, "Yeah, I've done this before, and last time was much harder." I grew up with a lot of privilege, but it didn't follow me out of Canada. In my early twenties, I was working for myself and paying my way. Now, because of that foundation, I feel like I'm unstoppable. I can do anything.

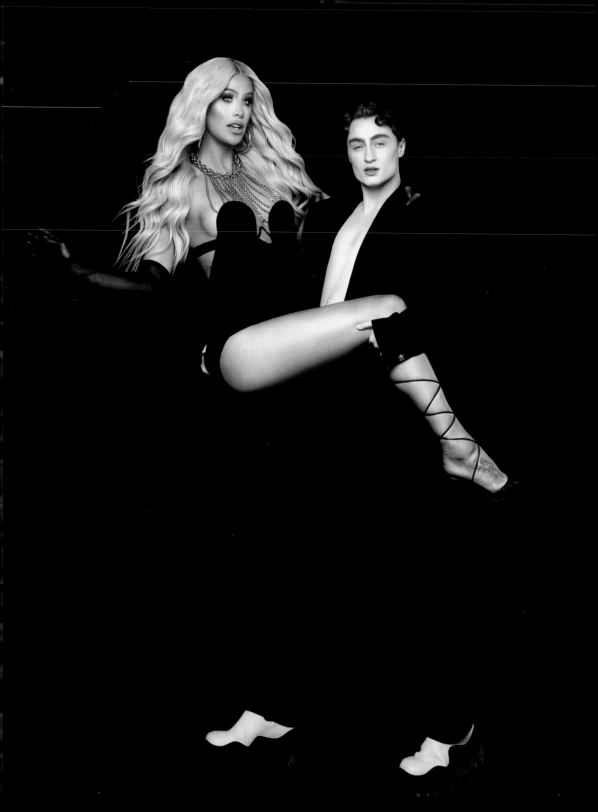

Gender Stereotypes & Dysphoria

For many people, transitioning highlights the intensity of gender as a social construct.

Everyone might be aware, to some degree, of how gender stereotypes affect them, but nobody understands this quite like trans people do. Who could possibly be more of an expert on gender constructs than people who have lived as more than one gender?

Frequently, in the beginning stages of transitioning, trans people feel the pressure to overcompensate with the goal of being read as more feminine or more masculine. How much of this is because they genuinely want to embody the gender they're stepping into, and how much of it is influenced by old-school beliefs about how men and women should behave? It can be confusing to untangle the personal from the societal, especially at the start of a transition.

Another major question about stereotypes is: will it always be this way? Right now, many societies are adopting a more fluid understanding of gender and sexuality, which might have an impact on how trans people see themselves and how the world sees them.

Speaking of how trans people see themselves, we're also going to talk about gender dysphoria in this section. In case you're new to that term, it refers to the discomfort that arises when a trans person feels the mismatch between their gender identity and their sex assigned at birth. For many people, gender dysphoria isn't something that disappears completely, but it does tend to get easier over time.

GIGI: Generally, I would say that for trans guys, there's a pressure to be masculine, and for trans girls, there's a pressure to be feminine.

GOTTMIK: Even to this day, it's rare to see any trans guys in the media who are not super macho. Sometimes I feel so alone within my own community because of how feminine I am, and I don't even really think I present that feminine in my day-to-day life out of drag. As I said before, I suppressed my transness for a while because I didn't fit in with the stereotypical hypermasculine model of a trans guy.

I should probably mention that there is a biological aspect to this, too. Testosterone is so much fiercer than estrogen, and it works faster. It takes over your body and changes it much more severely than estrogen does. Some trans guys who take testosterone end up looking pretty macho, but not everyone. That's just part of it.

GIGI: Do you feel like you've had to teach yourself to get louder?

GOTTMIK: I mean, I've always been a loud person, but I was absolutely socialized to be "girly" in other ways. Growing up, people would say things to me like, "Girls don't sit like that, girls don't wear that, girls don't do that." I have so many memories of just being frustrated.

The other thing was how it switched. As a little kid, all my friends were guys, and then when they started hitting puberty, suddenly they started treating me differently. They didn't want to just hang out. They wanted to hook up with me. It was so weird for me, because in my brain I was like, *I'm just one of the guys … and now I have to be careful around the guys.* For a while, it was just strange, and then I completely changed my role in the dynamic. Or, I guess you could say I leaned into the role they were giving me—hard.

If the guys were going to treat me like a girl, then I was going to become the most oversexualized, hyperfeminine girl in the world. And this is what I mean about being a naturally loud person. I've always loved being the center of attention. And I've always liked power. When I felt like my guy friends were trying to disempower me, I took all my power back and more. I started wearing these crazy wigs to school. I walked around like I owned everything. I was as out and proud as possible.

GIGI: I pretty much did the same thing! I went to a Catholic high school. When I started wearing makeup and leaning into a more flamboyant attitude, I would dress in the girl's uniform, which was a polo shirt and pants. The skirt had been phased out already. I would wear the tightest pants and the tightest polos and makeup on my face, and I quickly realized that the only way to avoid being bullied was to become a bully myself. I wasn't mean, but I was loud and confident and strong. I had to give everyone the impression that they shouldn't mess with me. It was a way to defend myself.

Then, after I started transitioning, I changed my demeanor. Stereotypically, loud girls are seen as obnoxious, or at least that's how I thought they were perceived, so I became quieter and more docile. When I moved to LA and started presenting myself in an even more feminine way, I made it a point to be extra sweet and small and all the things I thought a girly girl should be, but it just felt wrong to me. It wasn't my personality.

In situations that involved men, I liked playing the role of the girl to some degree. When a guy offered to pump my gas for me, for example, or opened the door for me, I'd think, *Oh good. I'm being seen as a woman and they're treating me like a woman.* Part of me liked it, and part of me didn't. I think before I was secure in myself as a woman, I was trying on different ways to be a "woman." And the first way I tried was to embody the stereotype of women as passive, and to buy into the most traditional version of gender roles. Now, if a guy wants to pump my gas or open the door for me, I think, *Oh, that's nice,* but I can also do that stuff for myself. I'm very independent, and at this stage in my journey, I don't need a guy treating me like a woman to feel like a woman.

GOTTMIK: Yeah, the change in how you're perceived when you switch genders is so crazy. Unlike cisgender people, trans people get to experience being stereotyped as two genders. I remember the first time I walked down the street looking like a guy, and a group of girls saw me and crossed the street. I thought, *What? I'm on your team! Don't worry!* But the truth is that women are taught to be wary of a guy walking by them in a hoodie at night, and for good reason. There are some creepy guys out there. But to be perceived as potentially one of them was such a trip for me, especially because in my mind, I looked so nonaggressive.

What I realized after that night was that I had to start treating girls differently. I had to factor in that they'd been taught not to trust men, just as I had, and act accordingly. Basically, I needed to go out of my way to present myself as a nonthreat in certain situations.

GIGI: Yes. It's crazy how differently you're treated when people think you're a man versus when they think you're a woman. Back in the day, when I was dressing as a girl, but not fully identifying as one yet, I'd go to the club in my makeup and be totally confident. I had no problem going up to people and starting a conversation. In my mind, I assumed that everybody thought I was a girl. But then, when the question would come up, I'd be like, "No, I'm a boy," and after that, I would be treated differently.

Later, when I started wearing extensions and taking the hormones and really identifying as a woman, I copied my friends' behavior. They were quiet and reserved, so I was, too—in public anyway. Behind closed doors, I was my natural loud self. Basically, if I had an audience, then I was performing the role of who I thought they wanted me to be.

I think it's important to point out that this happened almost subconsciously. Which speaks to how deeply ingrained our gender stereotypes are. Our roles are often just assumed without question. It took me years and years to start questioning how I was presenting myself, and what my beliefs were about gender roles. I really thought I had to fit into the cookie-cutter shape of a woman, and then, finally, I realized that no, I was allowed to be myself.

GOTTMIK: Right, but it's hard in the beginning, because the definition of "myself" is changing. Before I started transitioning, I loved dressing up like the "girliest" girl, as I said. Then, after my transition started, that changed. I thought I needed to hide my body, because my hips were too big and I had boobs. So I went from wearing cute dresses to living in baggy sweatpants, and this dramatic switch in my appearance had emotional consequences. I thought, *Well, if I'm living in baggy sweatpants, then who cares about how my hair looks.* I stopped putting energy into my appearance, which meant that I didn't look good, which meant that I didn't feel good about myself. What's crazy is that I didn't even connect the dots at the time. All I knew was that I felt sad.

Top surgery was a game changer, because I started dressing in the clothes I actually wanted to wear. Putting effort into my appearance made me feel cuter, and therefore better about myself, and eventually I got happier.

GIGI: Look good, feel better. Who doesn't feel better when they look amazing?

GOTTMIK: I think some people are less invested in their appearance and that's fine, but hello! I'm a makeup artist and a drag queen. I am very invested in appearances.

GIGI: You need to talk more about your makeup and drag life.

GOTTMIK: So, I started as a painter. Then I got into makeup, which is a similar art form, and I realized I was pretty good at it. In high school, I saw drag queens in our friend Marco Marco's fashion show, and I just thought it was the coolest thing ever. That was the first time I was really exposed to the world of drag.

After I moved to LA, I would do drag makeup on myself and go out in West Hollywood with a fake ID. I had so much makeup on that I literally could have been anyone, so nobody would question the ID. And then, once I got inside, everyone would assume that I was a guy in drag. It was the first time in my life I was ever confused for a guy.

And I loved it. I loved it so much that eventually, I refused to go out unless I was dressed in drag. I would go out with my best friend, Luna, who was a trans woman, in matching drag. We were like twins. Over time, I got better and better at drag, and I was exposed to a whole new community of queer people. When I started thinking about transitioning, I basically interviewed all of these people about their gender experiences. That's how I realized I was trans. And shortly after that, I became the first trans male contestant on *RuPaul's Drag Race*.

GIGI: Which meant that you were continuing to explore your gender and sexuality with an audience.

GOTTMIK: Yeah, I wasn't even completely out when I got on the show. My parents knew, and some friends, but my relatives had no idea. I was very much still in the process of getting comfortable with myself, and while I was on the show, my ideas about my sexuality changed, which was interesting. Before *Drag Race*, I always thought I was a gay guy. And then at some point I realized that if I was expecting people to see me for who I am, and not for what I decide or don't decide to do medically, then why wouldn't I have the same flexible ideas about everybody around me? It started to seem almost hypocritical to be romantically interested in only one gender. So, I realized I was pansexual, and it was freeing. I met so many amazing people. I'm still mostly interested in dating guys, but I'm open to meeting anyone.

GIGI: Exactly.

GOTTMIK: So, my understanding of my sexuality, my gender, and gender stereotypes in general has changed since I started my transition. And I would say that my relationship to dysphoria has changed, too.

GIGI: Please say more.

GOTTMIK: Before I transitioned, I was so dysphoric, but I couldn't pinpoint that at the time. I just thought I was just the most depressed person in the world. I would just wake up every morning and cry. I didn't even really know why.

And then when I started hormones, my mood changed. Hormones made me realize that I was on the right path, as I said before. It felt so good, and I wanted to keep chasing that good feeling. I thought that if I made more physical changes to my body, then I could eliminate any dysphoria that would ever happen.

What I've learned is that there's almost nothing, at least for me personally, that is going to take my dysphoria away. Every time I go to the bathroom at a club, it just triggers me. And then I often need a village to snap me back into reality, and even then, I rarely get back to the high vibe that I was at before I went to the bathroom. If something really misgendering happens in the middle of a fun night, I could easily spiral.

The conclusion I've come to is that dysphoria is something that will always be there. It's not always easy to deal with, but now I definitely have more of a comfort with who I am and a good, strong support system around me. I can bounce back now if something triggers my dysphoria. I just have to remember that even though it hurts, it's part of my journey as a human on this earth. All people go through hard things. When I put it into perspective like that, I feel a lot more confident that I can get through it.

GIGI: That word *dysphoria* has an "end of the world" vibe to it.

GOTTMIK: Right, but it doesn't have to be that way. Sometimes it doesn't affect me that much. If I see a picture of myself that doesn't match up with how I want to look, I just hit delete and move on.

GIGI: Same. I assume that I'll be having moments like that forever, but it doesn't stop me from living my life.

GOTTMIK: Many trans people experience dysphoria to some degree.

GIGI: A hundred percent.

GOTTMIK: Sometimes when I dress up in female drag, I will look at myself in the mirror and think, *This is too feminine*. Even though I'm literally doing female drag. Dysphoria is so pervasive. Sometimes I don't even realize how it's affecting me.

The reason I apply white makeup to my face sometimes when I do drag is because on certain days, seeing myself just as a gorgeous, feminine drag queen is just too much. I give myself a clown-white, alien look, which is anti-human and therefore anti-gender in a way.

GIGI: That's really interesting.

GOTTMIK: Yeah. And like we were saying before, I have to constantly check in to be sure that I'm making choices for me and not for other people. What I'm learning is that it's so important to let myself be fluid. Every day, I wake up and I'm in a different mood about gender. Sometimes I want to be more masculine, and other days I want to be more feminine.

GIGI: Right. And I think that within every gender identity, there's actually a nuanced spectrum. For me, it was just a matter of getting beyond the stereotype of what I thought a girl should be and finding my place on that spectrum.

GOTTMIK: Yes, and it's all subject to change, too. I mean, what is transitioning if not the constant state of change?

Follow Your Own Path

with Amanda Lepore

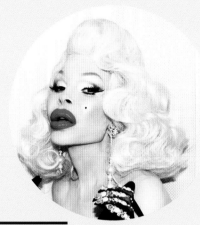

PHOTO BY **JOSEF JASSO**

My goal has always been to look as feminine as possible, but that doesn't mean my way is the right choice for everyone. We're all individuals, we all have different desires, and we need to respect each other's differences. However you choose to identify, and whatever you decide to do medically—hormones, no hormones; surgeries, no surgeries—you have to do for yourself. You're the one who has to be with yourself at the end of the day. Ultimately, it's all about self-love. If you love yourself, then you're going to be okay.

"If you love yourself, then you're going to be okay."

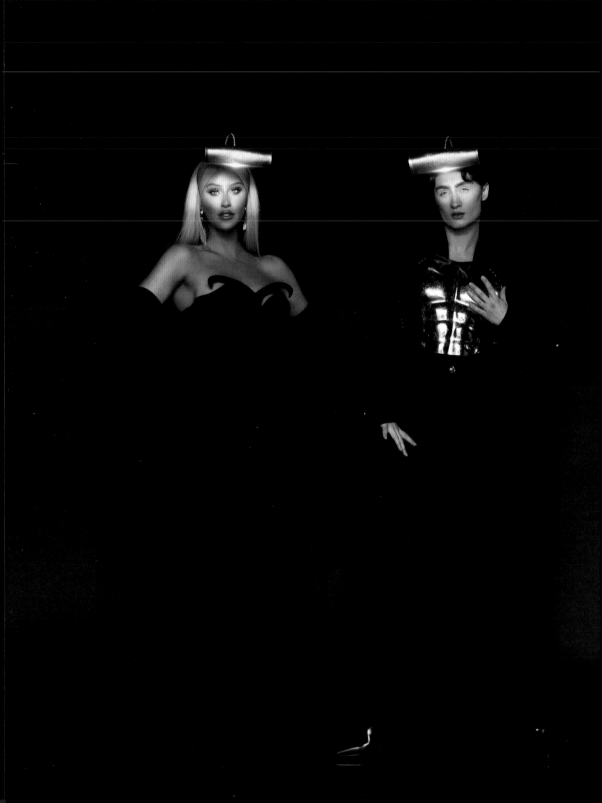

Role Models

Transitioning isn't easy, and you don't have to do it alone. Often, the natural first step is to find a role model in the media or in life who you want to emulate. Maybe somebody has the look you want, or the positive outlook on life. Ideally, at some point, you'll make a connection with a mentor online and/or in real life who can answer questions for you and give you a real sense of what it's like to live as a trans person. Having a support system around you makes a big difference.

GOTTMIK: Did you have any fashion role models you wanted to look like when you were younger?

GIGI: I just loved Victoria's Secret. Those models were my ideal. In high school, I would literally hack the computers in my art class so I could watch Victoria's Secret footage on YouTube. I was obsessed with Izabel Goulart, Alessandra Ambrosio, Tyra, and all the other girls. I was like, *Ah, that is what I want to look like.*

I also loved Sophia Loren so much that I named myself after her, as I mentioned before. I have so many memories of staring at the poster of her in my bedroom as a kid. I didn't know anything about her. I just knew that her face was so beautiful. She was a bombshell, and she definitely influenced my aesthetics.

GOTTMIK: Adam Lambert was huge to me. David Bowie was a big one, too. I was into anyone who was playing with gender in a fun way. Amanda Lepore was so major to me, as well. I remember seeing her when I was in 8th or 9th grade and being like, *Oh, she's taking what society thinks a woman should look like and hyperfeminizing it.* I was obsessed with how far she went. She looked like a blow-up doll or a David LaChapelle image. All the John Waters characters inspired me. I admired anyone who was taking reality and making it into whatever they wanted.

GIGI: Yes, that's how I felt about Betty, the trans girl I met when I was 19. It happened so randomly, now that I think about it. I was living in Toronto at the time, and my friend took me to a party in New York City where Betty happened to be working. I remember getting ready beforehand. I wore this American Apparel see-through lace dress, which was definitely lingerie, but I thought since it was New York City I could get away with it. Anyway, after the party, I met Betty and some of her friends, and I realized for the first time that I could live my life as a woman. I'd never met a trans woman before that night.

GOTTMIK: Did you know about Betty online before you met her?

GIGI: Yeah, and she became my ride or die. When I was coming out, I had my online support system, but in real life, it was Betty. I feel like it's so important to find one person to guide you. Maybe it's somebody who's a little older, or somebody who's a little ahead of you in the process. In the drag community, this person would be called a Drag Mom. In the trans community, it's a Trans Mom. I always called Betty my trans girlfriend, but I guess she was basically a Trans Mom.

GOTTMIK: Cute.

GIGI: Having her around gave me so much strength. She'd be like, "We got this. You are not alone." We were always making jokes to lighten the mood, which was huge, because being trans in public can be heavy at the beginning. I honestly don't know what I would have done without Betty. Before, in Toronto, I just wasn't meeting many trans people in the gay bars or gay clubs. I guess I got lucky, because I just happened to meet Betty at a party. I knew of trans people online, but meeting them in person allowed me to identify with them in a real way.

GOTTMIK: When I was thinking about transitioning, I didn't know any trans guys at all. I'd never even met one. So the internet was major for me. I found a few trans guys online who were posting their surgery and hormone results. Even though I didn't know them, just seeing their posts was so necessary for me. I just think the internet is the best resource ever, because you can watch videos and post comments. And you can contribute if you want. Remember when we filmed my top surgery and put it on your channel, Gigi?

GIGI: Of course.

GOTTMIK: And *Drag Race* is obviously available online, too. There's so much content to watch now, and it's a great way to connect with people. You can just start chatting.

I was looking at Reddit and TikTok recently, and there are pages of trans guys having conversations about *Drag Race* and being part of a little community. Going to the LGBTQ+ center in your area is another amazing thing to do, because there are so many people who are willing to help. Of course, so much of this depends on where you live. I feel like everyone's first step nowadays though is to do internet research. It's just so easy. And then, as far as in-person role models, you were definitely one of them, Gigi.

GIGI: I feel like finding someone who you vibe with is a big part of it. And we had a great vibe from the second we met.

GOTTMIK: Yes. You were perfect because you made it clear that you were definitely there for me, but you didn't pressure me. I just knew that I could ask you questions whenever I wanted, and that you'd give me room to think without pushing too much. You have this gift of making everything seem way more chill than it is, which honestly made every step of my transition so much easier. You helped me have the courage to come out and to say my name out loud and go on hormones and get surgery. And then there was that cute phase when we'd go to the doctor together and get shots together.

GIGI: It's so much more fun to do that stuff together. And it just normalizes the experience. In the beginning, if you go to lunch alone, or to the mall alone, it's a monumental and often scary thing. If you go to lunch with a trans friend, it's a lot less scary, and it also gives you reference. The next time you go to the mall, it doesn't seem so daunting because you've done it before.

GOTTMIK: Right, and if you get misgendered, your trans friend will have your back. Usually, during the day, I dress in a more masculine way, but sometimes, I'm in the mood to wear a heel and a crop top. Wearing this type of outfit to the mall in the daytime is very different from wearing it to a queer-friendly club at night, so I do have some anxiety about it, but also some excitement. I feel that it's a way of measuring how comfortable I've become, you know? It can feel really vulnerable, though, which is why it's much, much easier to do when I have trans friends with me.

GIGI: Yes.

GOTTMIK: And your configuration of role models can look however you want it to look, too. Along with my other trans friends and role models, I also have Violet Chachki, who calls herself my Drag Mom. She naturally stepped into that role and has taught me everything I know about the industry. She just brought me into the circle and gave me all her connections, which I really needed professionally when I first moved to LA and knew no one.

GIGI: I think it's easy to feel lost in the beginning, especially if you don't know any trans people. As Gottmik was saying before, the internet is a fabulous resource. If you see someone online who you admire, write to them. Be proactive. Ask them questions. Ask them if they'll be your Trans Mom. A lot of people love taking on that role and are more than happy to help guide you.

GOTTMIK: Exactly. If you're obsessed with someone online, figure out a way to meet them. The first step to finding your tribe is envisioning your tribe.

GIGI: You have to manifest it.

"The first step to finding your tribe is envisioning your tribe."

GOTTMIK: Yes. You have to keep manifesting your ideal situation and eventually, you'll get it. It's normal nowadays to write to people online.

GIGI: Right. Just don't be a creeper about it.

GOTTMIK: And find people who are doing what you're doing. If you're a musician, make connections with musicians. If you're a designer, find other designers.

GIGI: And in the meantime, stay focused on your own life and your own passions. Find what makes you happy.

GOTTMIK: If whatever you're doing is not making you happy, then it's time to move on and try something else. Sometimes, you have to figure out what works by figuring out what doesn't work.

GIGI: Yes, and if all of this sounds like a lot, just know that things do eventually shift. You will find your role models if you look for them, and you will find your trans friends.

GOTTMIK: You will. And then later, you'll become somebody's role model. That's the amazing thing about the community. You get to pay it forward.

Show Up

with Violet Chachki

As a Catholic student growing up, I was seemingly the only boy getting uniform violations because I wanted to wear something other than khaki slacks every day. It seemed as though the girls were given many more options to express themselves, and I wanted that too. Instead, the idea of boys expressing themselves this way was always looked down on. But as a rebellious person, if I'm told not to do something, I'm going to do it. "No" might be my favorite word, but that doesn't mean I like to hear it!

I stole women's clothing from thrift stores, played dress-up when home alone, and even went as an Olsen twin for Halloween one year. Turns out, I got a lot of attention for the costume, and it felt great! I had only ever felt negativity from people for expressing myself, so this positive attention became very addictive. Soon after, I entered the world of drag and never looked back.

Starting any new stage in one's life is going to be hard, especially for a queer person learning just who they are and finally allowing themself to express that loudly and proudly. Without the right support, it's basically impossible. Too often, this support won't come from the families they were born into. Any queer person will tell you just how important it is to find your chosen family—people you bring into your life who see you, hear you, understand you, and support you. Never have I met someone as aligned with my approach to everything from my drag career to my personal interests and opinions as Gottmik. He is my chosen family. And with all the positive and negative lessons I've learned over the years, whether in terms of show business, drag, or life in general, I try to be the best role model I can be. I never want him to go through the hardships I did.

It's not always about who has the most experience or success—it's about showing up, no matter what.

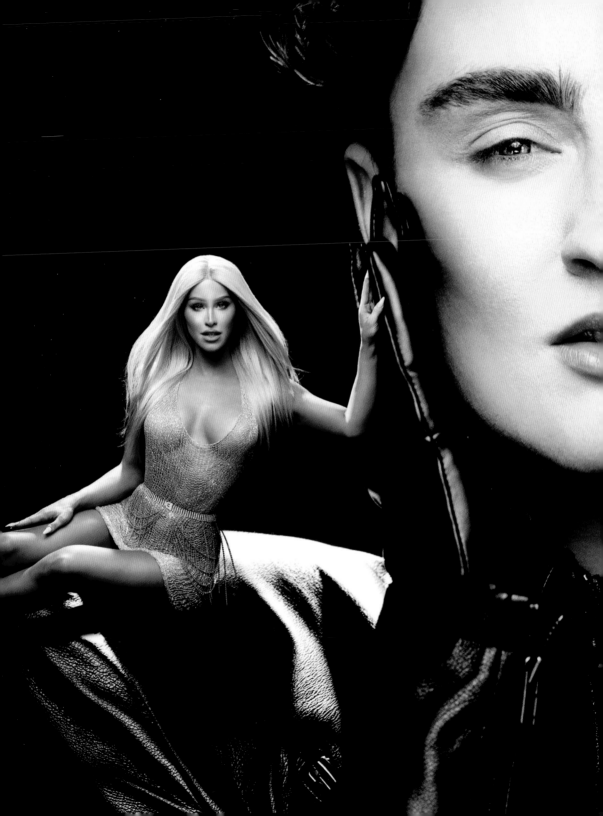

Tips for Looking Masculine or Feminine

We want to make tons of room for fluidity in this conversation and being fluid often includes a reconceptualization of the words *masculine* and *feminine* when it comes to appearance—and everything else.

It's also true that many trans people (including us) are interested in the far sides of the masculine/feminine spectrum. That's because we, like a lot of trans guys and girls, feel most like ourselves when our appearance is accentuated to match our gender.

GIGI: We often make assessments about whether a person is masculine or feminine based on a bunch of features, and some of them are more key than others. When you're trans, you're kind of forced to become an expert on human anatomy, and you get really familiar with all the little tricks you can use so that people are more likely to perceive you (and you're more likely to perceive yourself) in the way that you want.

GOTTMIK: Which tip should we start with?

GIGI: Oh! I just learned a hand trick for veins.

GOTTMIK: Oh, veins are a thing.

GIGI: Okay, so when you leave your hands down by your sides for a long time, all the blood goes down there.

GOTTMIK: And it makes your veins look bigger.

GIGI: Right. But if you put your hands up in the air and shake them for like 10 seconds, the veins become less pronounced and your hands look softer. If somebody's wanting to take a picture at the club, I like to do a little shake-the-hands-dance before posing.

GOTTMIK: And then for guys, it's the opposite.

GIGI: Right, you swing your arms around to send all the blood to your hands.

GOTTMIK: And the veins in your hands and in your arms become instantly more visible. If I take a photo right after I do this, people look at it and are often like, "Oh my God, your arms."

GIGI: What's another trick?

GOTTMIK: Height's a big one. I would say definitely get some insoles if you want to be taller.

GIGI: Do you do that?

GOTTMIK: I started to in Europe because I was around all these models and in pictures, I looked so short in comparison and I hated it. So, I bought some insoles and now I think they're everything. I wear them in all my shoes. Seriously, you just slide them in and it's game over.

GIGI: I think height's a huge one for girls, too. Because it's like, if you see a very tall, built girl walking down the street, you either think she's a supermodel or you think she's a man. So, either you wear your high heels anyway and you own it, or you buy some shoes with a lower heel if that makes you more comfortable.

GOTTMIK: You kind of have to understand the proportions of the body, though. So, if your rib cage is longer, you need to know where you should be cinching. The same wisdom can be applied to feet. If you have a bigger foot, it needs to have a higher arch, because then it'll look smaller. Girls who wear a lower heel have almost no arch, so their feet look longer. I feel like if you're tall and it's a night for heels, you might as well go full-on glamazon and get some gorgeous high high heels with a serious arch.

GIGI: I feel a lot of girls make mistakes with the footwear.

GOTTMIK: All the time. So many girls think a little kitten heel is the way to go, but actually, it does the feet no favors.

GIGI: Whereas if you wear a very high heel, people just go, "Oh, gorgeous."

GOTTMIK: Being in the drag world, I've really learned how to proportionize a body and it's so important to remember that what works for one person may not work for you. I need a completely different corset shape than most of my friends because I happen to have a smaller torso. It really depends on your particular body type.

GIGI: Right. Another one for girls is tucking. I didn't know what this was until I saw my friends using tucking undergarments. I was like, "Excuse me, what is that?" I went online to search for them, and all I could find at the time was a brand that was marketed for crossdressers. I ordered five and they worked, but they were too thick. I eventually found a better brand, and I love tucking now. Every single time I go out, I tuck. It just makes me feel cute.

GOTTMIK: For guys it's packing, which gives the illusion that you have a dick. Basically, you buy a silicone dick and put it in your pants. My personal opinion on this is that it's best to go smaller than you think you need to. I know that when a lot of people start out, they try a 5- or 6-inch dick, which is which is a bit large for when it's supposed to be soft. Smaller is more realistic. You can even buy ones now with pubes on them.

GIGI: Oh, that's everything.

GOTTMIK: There are so many different ways to attach it. I have some friends who tie it around themselves and others who glue it on. And then there are ones that allow you to stand while you're peeing, which is a game changer, because bathrooms are a whole thing for trans people.

GIGI: A whole thing.

GOTTMIK: Yes. And there are a ton of makeup tricks for guys who are into that. Let me tell you a fun story about how I learned one of them. It happened at David LaChapelle's house. Yes, David LaChapelle's house. If you had told me when I was a teenager in Arizona that I would be doing a photo shoot at David LaChapelle's house, I would have died.

             Anyway, David LaChapelle told me he wanted the guys to look really natural, and like they were blushing. He said, "Like this," and then he put some blush on his finger and started at the apple of his cheek and pulled downward. I hadn't thought of it before, but guys do blush in a lower place than girls. I use that tip when I do my makeup now, and then I apply bronzer, also in a downward motion.

GIGI: Wow, I love that!

GOTTMIK: The main trick with makeup and guys is to apply everything really lightly, because if you're going for a masculine look, you probably don't want people to know you're wearing makeup at all. Be light-handed. A little makeup can go a long way.

GIGI: I love doing my lips, because that's what people look at when you're speaking. The lip lift really helped feminize my face, and I accentuate my lips even more with lipstick. Everything on girls is placed slightly differently than on guys. As you just said, Gottmik, blush placement is different. The lash placement is also different. Brows are a huge thing. Hair is a huge thing. I have a few easy hairstyles I do when I want to read as female and I don't have a ton of time.

GOTTMIK: Remember how before you got your hairline surgery, I used to pencil in a rounded hairline for you?

GIGI: I forgot about that.

GOTTMIK: That was major.

GIGI: Major.

GOTTMIK: And then obviously, there are binders for guys. I remember when I got my first one, it was the happiest day of my life. I was obsessed. I bought so many of them.

GIGI: It looks kind of like a sports bra, right?

GOTTMIK: Yes, but the front is made of thicker material. Binders are so uncomfortable, but the effect is amazing. One important thing that a lot of guys ignore is that you're only supposed to wear them for 6 to 8 hours. It can be dangerous if you keep them on longer than that. Just make sure your body's going to be okay.

GIGI: When you do something uncomfortable for long enough, the discomfort becomes your normal and it's easy to forget that your body isn't happy.

GOTTMIK: Right, it just becomes a habit.

GIGI: I love thinking about you in the moment you put on your first binder and thought, *Oh, yes*.

GOTTMIK: Oh my God. I still have a video of it. I remember I turned to the side and posed. I was so excited. The binder changed my attitude, and so did a lot of these tricks.

GIGI: A little can go a long way.

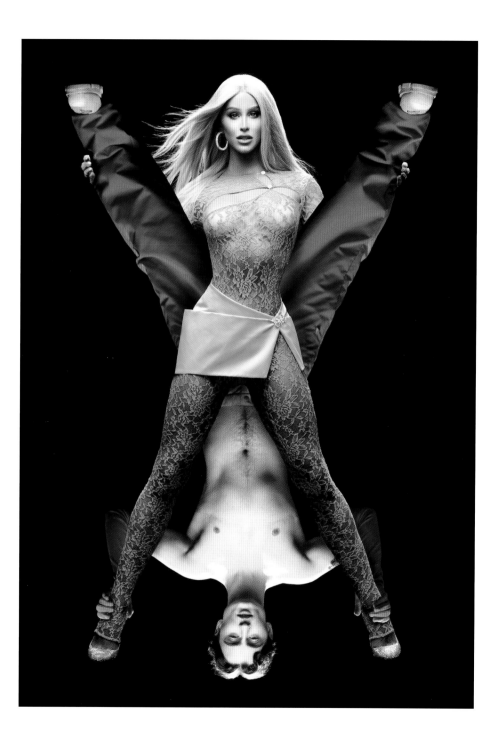

Gottmik's Masculinization Tips

Here are some tips on how to feel more masculine and comfortable in your body. Although these methods worked for me, they may not all be right for you. It will take some trial and error to find what gives you what you're looking for.

FACE

Jaw: The very first thing that helped me with facial dysphoria was squaring everything out. I was able to do that with the help of filler. I put a bit in my chin and then I put a generous amount toward the back of my jaw to create a more angular, 90 degree look.

Brow: Since I don't have a protruding brow bone, I also use a bit of Botox to lower the front of my brow and snatch up the ends, taking away a bit of lid space.

Makeup: When doing my makeup, I like to add a bit of tinted moisturizer to even everything out but not take away 100 percent of my natural skin tone and texture. Then I suck in my cheeks and apply a bit of bronzer down my cheekbone and down by my mouth to accentuate that sunken cheekbone look. I also love to take the bronzer and contour my jaw a bit more.

Eyebrows: I wanted to have a bit of a thicker brow look as well, so I got a masculinizing micro blade, which is basically a cosmetic tattoo to add a bit of volume and shape to your eyebrows.

Hair: Getting your first haircut after you may have had long hair can be so scary. Do not ask me why but to this day going into a barber shop and getting my hair cut will make me anxious. The key is knowing your face shape and what you want to achieve with your hair. There are amazing websites that have every face shape possible and give suggestions for the best result. I think the best tip overall is to make sure everything is angular. For a while I was just getting my hair cut short but not lining up the sides and forehead so it wasn't really giving me the masculine look I was looking for. No matter what hair I'm rocking (mullet, pompadour, buzzed, you name it!), I want to create square angles.

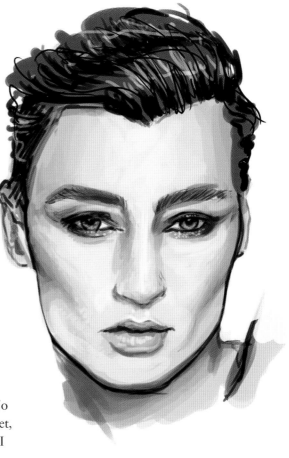

BODY

Chest: Top surgery was such a major dysphoria relief for me. Make sure you find a doctor who works with you and can achieve the type of top surgery that is correct for you! If you get a double incision like I did, make sure you're vocal about what shape you want the scars to be and work with the doctor so you end up with your dream chest.

Scars: I love my top surgery scars, but since I have a lot of red undertones, I wanted to tone down the redness a bit. I tried lasers, but for me, scar camouflage ended up being the best option. This includes basically tattooing your scars with a skin tone.

Binders: Top surgery isn't cheap, and surgery isn't an easy or fun thing. So, if you're living in a space that you're not completely out or supported, it may not be possible yet. When that was my case, binding my chest was a huge help to me. I cried when I got my first binder because it truly was the first time I felt like I was taking steps to transition the way I wanted! gc2b is a trans POC [person of color]-owned business that has some of the best binders on the market, in my opinion. Please remember to research how to bind safely, as it can be very dangerous. I do know people who have felt so dysphoric they've had to sleep in them and ended up getting hurt.

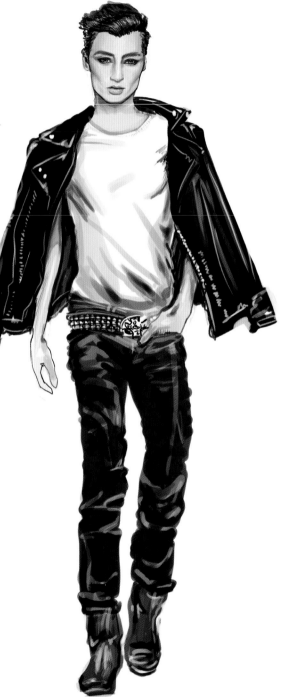

STP: Using an STP (or stand to pee prosthetic) really changed the game for me as well! I never really had bottom dysphoria when clothed, but the second I had to pee in certain settings, it made me a bit anxious (which is insane typing this out because everyone pees, but I'm just being honest here no matter how embarrassing it may be). STPs gave me a bit of bulk and made using any bathroom a breeze. And trust me, no matter how much bathroom anxiety you get, no one is looking. My favorite prosthetic is from a brand called Reelmagik. They make insanely realistic prosthetics and have mastered every functionality you could think of! It's not the cheapest thing in the world, but they do have payment plans. This is definitely something that would be hard to get if you're living with parents or a place where you're not totally out, which was a huge reason I didn't have one for so long. However, LGBTQ+ centers can be great resources to obtain some of these gender-affirming items.

Abs and Waist: Focusing on working out my side abs really helped bulk out my waist and square out my body. I obviously love a tiny, cinched waist in drag, but my hips sometimes make me feel a bit dysphoric. Working out the side of my body was really the best thing to help me with this.

Arms: Testosterone really helped make the veins in my arms more pronounced, which I love! But if hormones aren't for you, you can also pump out your veins by working out your arms.

Body Hair: Growing out my body hair really helped my dysphoria, and I also noticed I don't get misgendered as much if I have facial or body hair.

Height: Trust me, we love short kings. We really do. But sometimes, being the only guy not over six feet isn't my favorite thing, so I started wearing boots with a bit of a platform (not technically platform boots but something more than a totally flat shoe) with lifts inside to give me an extra couple inches when I'm feeling the discomfort.

Outfits: I always wanted to hide my body with baggy clothing, but I've learned wearing an outfit or silhouette that works for your body type is a way better option. There are so many amazing resources online to find what looks will square out your body and give you the shape you're looking for!

Gendered Clothing: Don't be scared off by gendered clothing! Gender is a spectrum, and sometimes the jacket in the women's section may give you the look you want. I wasted so much time thinking I had to only shop in the men's section but that is so not true. Fashion is for everyone!

Gigi's Feminization Tips

Here are some makeup and accessory tips I find helpful when it comes to feeling confidently feminine. I recommend experimenting to find your own style and preferences.

Brows: This depends on your natural growth and preference, of course, but thinning the brow can soften the face and dramatically transform it instantly!

Lashes: Lashes decorate the windows to the soul and instantly make you look more flirtatious and accentuate the beautiful shape of your eyes!

Eyes: Keep the waterline clean, because it'll keep your eyes open and GORGEOUS! You can even apply a light nude waterline to open them up even more!

Cheekbones: Blush is always a good idea when applied high on the cheekbones. Cream highlight on the cheekbones adds a glow!

Lips: Overline with lip liner in the center only to lift the upper lip and give you a pout. A glossy lip is always beautiful and SO girly!

Makeup: Remember, less is MORE! Make sure the facial hair and skincare are on point, and use a light hand when applying foundation and contour.

Face: Bronze/warm up the perimeter of the entire face in order to minimize the forehead, jaw, and chin while carving in the cheekbone. Don't forget to blend!

Hair: If you're wearing a lace front [wig], pull it down to make your face look smaller and more feminine.

Earrings: Little studs or hoops do a world of wonder for framing the face and adding a little sparkle.

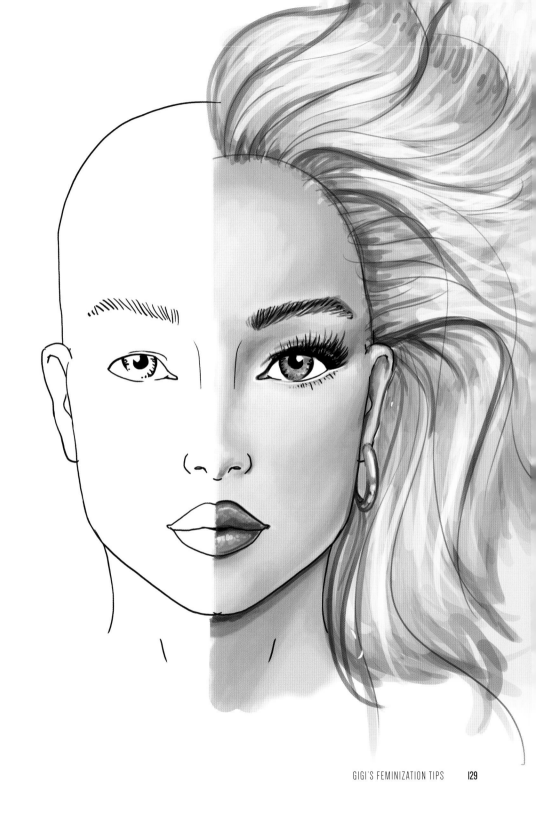

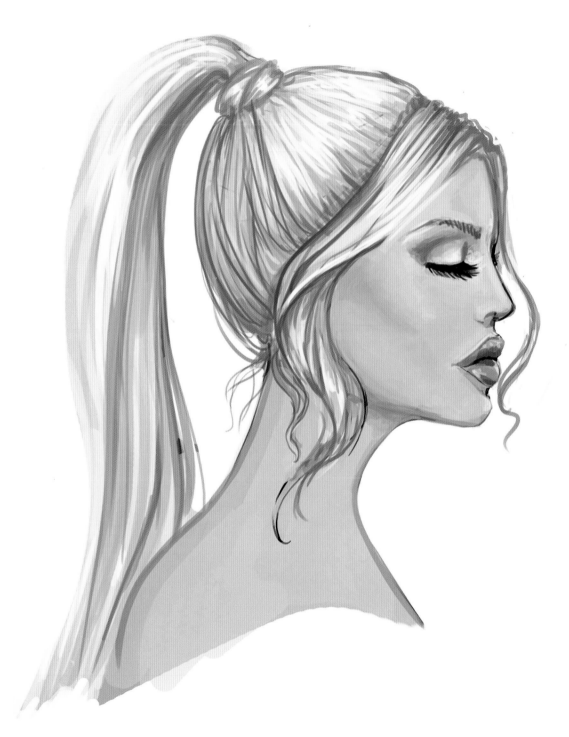

Paris Hilton's *Guide to*
Being Confidently Feminine

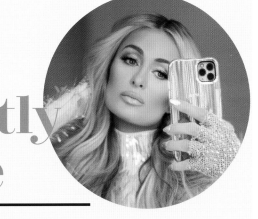

PHOTO BY **BRENDAN FORBES**

- Share your inner sparkle with the world by incorporating glitter into your fashion rotation. This is your time to shine.

- Don't shy away from classically beloved frills like lace and ribbons—after all, you're a gift to this world so you might as well put a bow on it.

- Never underestimate the power of a little lip gloss to give you that extra touch of irresistible seduction.

- Get a crisp, bright manicure to ensure you're manifesting your inner beauty even on your fingertips. You can never go wrong with pink.

- Tantalize everyone you encounter through voluminous hair. There's nothing I love more than timelessly wavy locks.

- Embrace high heels because you can climb every mountain and you can do it in style.

- Wear outfits that make you feel completely unstoppable and unapologetically you. The world is your runway.

- And last, but certainly not least, my most important boss babe tip: be confident, because there's nothing more beautiful than believing in yourself. As I would say, *that's hot*.

Gigi's
Cautionary Silicone Tale

I want to share something I've never shared before out of fear of shame and judgment. I'm not proud of this cautionary tale.

Many years ago, my friend (let's call her Veronica) invited me to a pumping party. What is a pumping party? Basically, someone takes a syringe full of silicone and injects it into your butt, your hips, your thighs—wherever you need a little bit more volume. Veronica assured me that it was totally safe and sterile and that the results would look completely natural. It was hospital-grade silicone, she said. The only catch was that it would be injected secretly in a hotel room by someone who wasn't a doctor, which was illegal.

Part of me was scared, but another part of me was like, *What could go wrong?* Veronica and other girls I knew had had it done, and they had survived. Veronica lived in New York City, so I scheduled the procedure into one of my trips there.

On the day of the procedure, I was nervous, but Veronica quelled my nerves. Just as I was feeling at ease, the phone rang. It was Lisa at the front desk.

A few minutes later, she was in our room, covered in tats and carrying a Coach bag that was bursting at the seams with her medical equipment. What was Lisa's official title? Trainer. If someone complimented you after a procedure, the thing to say was, "Oh, thanks, I just went to the trainer." (Wink wink.) Another important thing to know about Lisa: her ass was bigger than any ass I had ever seen in real life. It looked so overdone, which was not exactly reassuring.

Lisa locked the door behind her and laid out all her materials: gauze, syringes, silicone. As she poured our doses of silicone, I noticed it seemed a little liquid-y. When I voiced my concern, I was reassured by Lisa and Veronica that it was okay.

Veronica went first. She was in so much pain once Lisa began the injections. Lisa would close each injection hole with super glue and a Band-Aid. "Keep this on for at least twenty-four hours so that the silicone stays in," she said.

Sketchy? Yes. For the fifth or sixth or hundredth time, I thought about abandoning this crazy mission. But then, somehow, I was lying on the bed and biting my forearm just like Veronica had. The needle was thick, which increased the pain, but what I mostly felt was pressure. I didn't know exactly where the silicone was being injected, but Lisa assured me it was in very strategic spots.

Now, years later, I've heard countless horror stories of girls dying during procedures like this, because the "trainer" injected the silicone in the wrong place, which I didn't know at the time. All I knew was that after the procedure was done, and the results looked so good. I felt feminine and beautiful and like all the sketchiness had been worth it.

That night, we went to a big hangout for trans girls at that time. I ran into a friend and excitedly told her about my experience. I lifted up my dress to show her the amazing results—but my friend was worried for me. "Girl, if you got that done today, then you should be at home resting right now."

I freaked out after that. I wanted the silicone out of me. So I went to the bathroom, peeled off my Band-Aids, picked off the super glue, and sat down on the toilet seat to push it out. When I stood up, the floor was slicked with silicone. I tiptoed out, grabbed another cocktail, and decided to forget the whole thing.

Months went by, and then Veronica hit me up again with another pumping party offer with Lisa. I still don't understand why, but I said yes.

The scene in the hotel room the second time was like déjà vu. Eventually, Lisa appeared and I was getting injected again—with even more silicone than the last time because that's how it works. Every session, your body can tolerate a little more, and I, again, was happy with the results. I left the silicone in this time.

Now, looking back, I can see how I completely ignored my gut instinct to flee those hotel rooms. I was ready to do whatever it took to be as feminine as possible—at the cost of my own comfort and well-being. My advice about pumping parties? Don't do them. Seek professional medical help. Keep yourself safe. If you feel sketched out, leave.

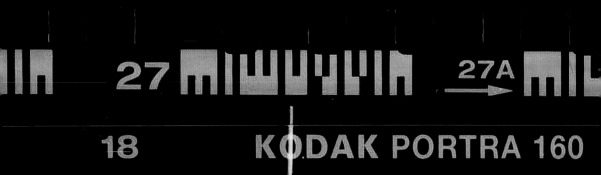

27 27A

18 KODAK PORTRA 160

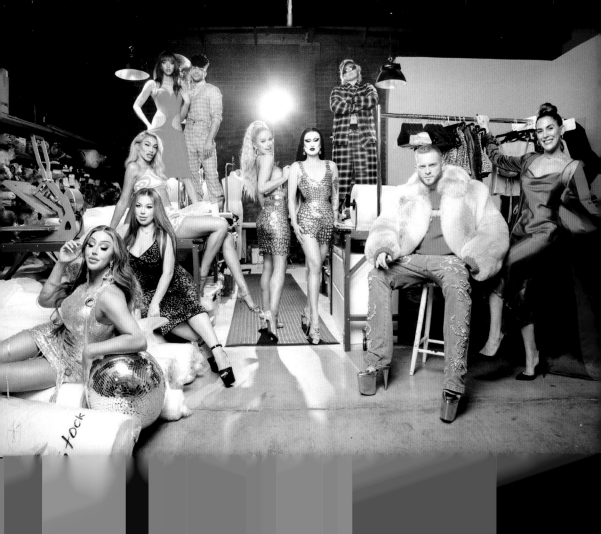

28   28A →

19   KODAK PORTRA 1

PART 3

YOUR NEW LIFE

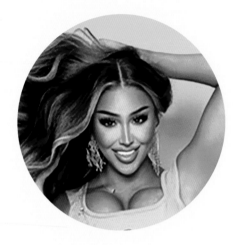

La Demi Martinez *on*

Staying Safe

PHOTO BY **CHRIS MARTIN**

My story begins in an underground club in Los Angeles, where I had met a cute guy and we were hitting it off. While hanging out, this cute guy (let's call him Sam) said he had a friend on the way. Soon after, a very tall gay man whom I recognized from events around town walked into the club. This was Sam's friend. Seeing me and Sam together, he beelined over and split us up. We weren't sure what the problem was but we ignored him and hooked up the rest of the night.

Although Sam and I lost touch over the next few months, I ran into him at a house party one night. We decided to hook up again and, after we split up to meet at his car, I ran into his friend

on the staircase. He told me Sam didn't want me and knocked me on the side of the head. I fell and he continued to beat me, he de-wigged me, and he dragged me down the stairs, my bag spilling my things everywhere. He ran off after threatening to attack me again the next time he saw me.

That night, I posted everything I knew about the incident and my attacker, and social media took over the next day. My attacker was publicly recognized but continued to attend events and make appearances without any questioning. I soon learned the hard way that I was seemingly on my own. Nobody from the party came forward, and the police dragged their feet in assigning anyone to my case. To this day, nothing has happened and I'm considered a liar by some, even with evidence in my favor.

Would the police have behaved differently if I'd been a cis woman? It's hard not to imagine that the answer to that question is yes. What makes the story even worse is that my attacker is a gay man, advocating to his millions of followers that he is a supportive member of the queer community.

What I learned from this atrocious incident is how important it is to protect yourself. If I could give any trans girl advice, I would say be careful, and don't assume that others, even when they appear to be allies, have your best interests at heart. It's a ruthless world out there for us girls, and I am a prime example as to why you should always look over your shoulder. My wounds may have healed, but the trauma will live with me for the rest of my life. He deserves to be behind bars. I don't care how long it takes, but justice will be served before he has the chance to do worse to someone else.

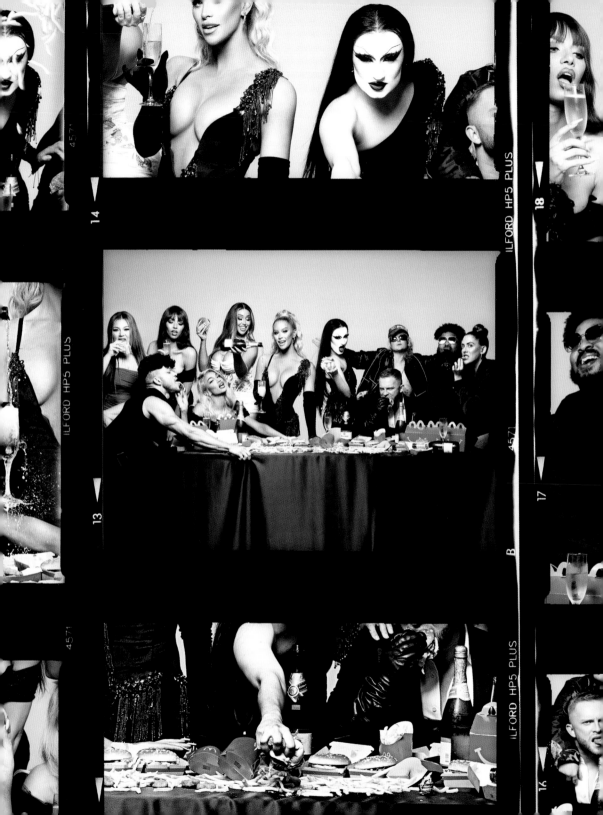

Chosen Family

Building a strong community is a vital part of life for many queer individuals. What this looks like is different for everyone. A common misconception is that having a chosen family means you've excommunicated your biological family. This might be the case, but it definitely doesn't have to be. All that matters is that you have a group of people around you who are trustworthy and supportive.

GOTTMIK: Chosen family is truly the most important thing in the world to me. I know I wouldn't have been able to transition as fiercely as I did without them. As I said before, I didn't know any trans people before I moved to LA. And then I got here, and there were trans women all around me. I felt very lucky to be surrounded by all of these amazing girls who helped to show me the way. Even though my transition was different from theirs, we were bonded by our transness.

GIGI: Same. If I hadn't had my trans family, it would have been so much harder. I think that seeing trans people online is one thing, and then actually meeting them is the next step. It makes you feel like you really belong.

GOTTMIK: Exactly. You can watch YouTube videos and do research, which is great, but hanging with another trans person is everything.

GIGI: It really is.

GOTTMIK: What's interesting is that I didn't find any trans men I identified with at the beginning, and I still haven't really found them. Even now, when I go out, I don't really meet trans guys.

GIGI: Honestly, it's mostly women at the places we go to.

GOTTMIK: Right. I can definitely count all the trans guys I know in Los Angeles on one hand.

GIGI: I feel that a lot of trans guys are romantically interested in women, so after they transition they are heterosexual. And that's why they're not at the gay bars we go to.

GOTTMIK: True. I definitely have been able to meet some amazing trans men while traveling, and I would love to see more of us out here loud and proud! On the other hand, while this is a stereotype, trans girls seem more visible because many of them often love being pretty and validated for their appearances.

GIGI: How trans women are seen in the queer community might play a role, too. We are held on the highest level. If you're a trans girl at the gay bar, you are the doll, you are the diva; it's basically your club. There's a ton of opportunity to meet amazing trans women friends in the queer scene, whereas a lot of trans guys don't really identify with the queer scene. Maybe they feel like they don't belong. Do you think that's true?

GOTTMIK: Maybe. Recently, I've been meeting more trans guys who identify as gay, so it might be changing.

GIGI: Right. I think another important thing to mention when it comes to forming your community is that every relationship is a lesson. Don't put all your eggs in one basket, because people will burn you. It takes a minute to get to know people. That's just part of life. If you cast a wide net, then you're less likely to be disappointed. I think expecting to find all the best people right out of the gate is highly unlikely. It takes a little time to build your chosen family.

GOTTMIK: It took me five years of living in LA before I felt like I'd found my people, and now it's so good. I can leave town and not talk to members of my chosen family for a while, and I know that when I get back, they'll all be here. My relationships feel solid in that way now. It's comfortable and cute.

GIGI: And strongly encouraged.

GOTTMIK: Definitely.

GIGI: The other thing I want to add is that even when a friendship dies, it's not necessarily a loss. Not all relationships need to go on forever. Sometimes, really important ones last for a finite amount of time. Eventually, you might outgrow one another or realize you have irreconcilable differences, but that doesn't mean the friendship was necessarily bad. Maybe it caused you to realize something important about yourself. Maybe it made you a stronger person. I would not be where I am today without Betty, for example, but now we don't talk anymore. And that's okay. But she taught me so much, and I would not exchange that time for the world.

GOTTMIK: Right. I think chosen family changes over time.

GIGI: The more you get to know yourself, the more you understand what you need, and that impacts your relationships.

GOTTMIK: Yes. What you need is always changing.

GIGI: I feel we need to mention, too, that having a chosen family doesn't necessarily mean you're excommunicating your family. For a lot of people, it does mean that, but it doesn't have to. It depends on how accepting your biological family is of your transness.

GOTTMIK: In the best-case scenario, it's nice to have a chosen family in addition to your biological one. Even if your parents are the most loving people in the world, they're never going to understand what you're going through on an experiential level. They just can't. Which means that even if they want to help you, they can only help you to a certain degree, and some of them don't even know where to begin. A lot of parents worry that your life is going to be full of obstacles, which isn't exactly uplifting when you're trying to transition.

GIGI: You need people around you who are in the community.

GOTTMIK: Yes, and that can include anyone under the queer umbrella. Whether you're trans, gay, pan, or whatever else, we're all standing on common ground. We all know what it was like to grow up queer and feel like we didn't belong. And many of us probably had to deal with the heterosexuality that permeated our childhoods, sometimes in the form of offensive décor choices. I had to grow up with a sea-themed bathroom, for example. I feel like being a queer child with artistic abilities in a land of heterosexuals just isn't talked about enough, honestly.

GIGI: Hetero people can have chosen families, too, obviously, but for queer people, who are often oppressed for their sexuality, it's extra important.

GOTTMIK: Right. For a lot of queer people, they need a chosen family in order to survive, and for a lot of straight people, it's an elective thing. They're not fighting for their rights in the same way we are.

GIGI: Yes. I think it's incredibly hard when people have a family that's unaccepting and live in a place that doesn't value queerness. For those people, going online is probably the best way to start building a community.

"In the best-case scenario, it's nice to have a chosen family in addition to your biological one."

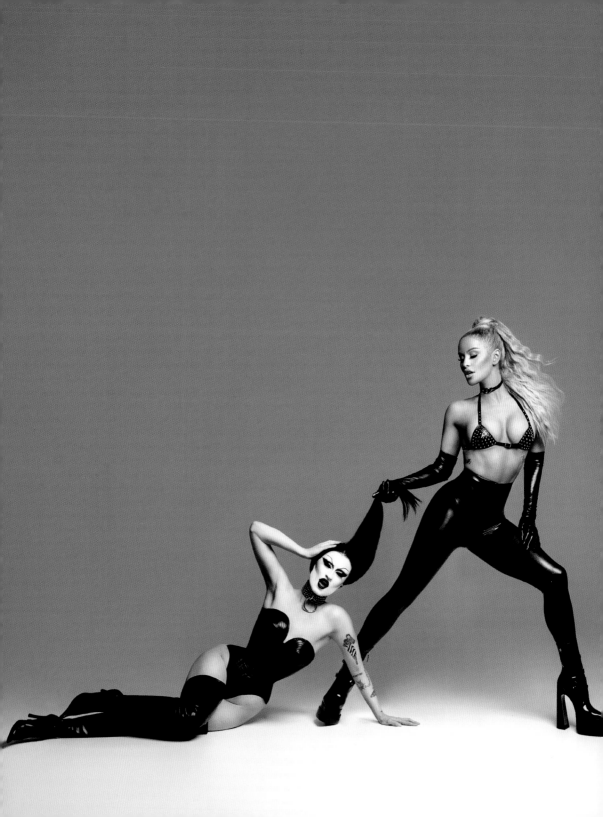

Competition Within the Community

Unfortunately, competition exists everywhere, and the trans community is no exception. It's natural to look at someone and admire their features, their personality, and/or their success, but feeling like you're in competition with that person can be toxic. Instead of allowing other people to make you feel less than, use them as inspiration. Remember that the pictures you see on social media aren't necessarily authentic. (Hello, Facetuning.) And most importantly, when you feel the competitive vibes taking over, remind yourself that if we want to make progress as a community, we're going to do it a lot faster and more healthily if we all stick together.

GOTTMIK: I think we should start with you telling the Betty story.

GIGI: The short version is that after I got to know her better, I noticed a red flag or two. But because she was so important to me, I kind of just chose to ignore them. At some point during our friendship, she became close with my manager, Scott. He's been my manager since the very beginning when I was nobody, but we did go through this tough period where I felt like we were growing apart. During that time, Betty came to LA to stay with me. One day, we went to lunch and I confided in her. I told her that I felt like Scott and I were no longer friends. It was just all business.

            Flash forward to a few days later: she wasn't in the apartment. Because she was out to lunch. With Scott. Saying not nice things about me and telling Scott he should represent her instead, I later learned.

GOTTMIK: Insane.

GIGI: I immediately thought, *Oh no, what else did I tell her?* She ended up leaving, and Scott and I had a big conversation. We're still together. I never talked to Betty after that day.

GOTTMIK: She fully just tried to swoop in and take what you had.

GIGI: It was a hard lesson. I was young, maybe 21 or 22, and she was my first trans girlfriend, so I held her in such high regard. Unfortunately, there's a lot of competition in the trans female community. A lot of us feel so much emptiness within our hearts, and we're starved for validation. Many of those who don't have it will do anything to get it. If they see somebody doing better than they're doing and they don't feel fulfilled within themselves, they can get mean. Back then, I might have wanted more professional accolades than I had, but even so, I was happy. And I would never have hurt anybody. I don't think happy people hurt people. It doesn't work that way.

            Of course, this applies to humans in general, but there's a specific brand of savagery within the trans female community. It can be cutthroat. This may sound depressing to somebody who's new to being trans and feeling anxious in general, but I still think it's worth saying: you have to be careful about you who trust, especially when you're in the vulnerable position of changing genders. You have to be guarded. And it would be great to not ignore red flags like I did.

GOTTMIK: What I love is that you're not jaded by that experience. You just got smarter.

GIGI: Thank you. I definitely didn't shut down and not let people in after that. I'm still really open. I might even be too open sometimes. As you know, Gottmik, my friends and my husband sometimes have to tell me that someone is bad news. I don't see it. I usually wait until I get burned to cut someone off, which is both good and bad. I really do see the best in people. But I don't forget being burned. Once it's over, it's over.

GOTTMIK: I'm prone to cutting people off, maybe with a quickness that's sometimes unfair. When my parents weren't being a hundred percent accepting in the beginning, I cut them off for a minute, which was unnecessary. I've been scarred by a lot of bad relationships, though, so if I see a red flag, I sprint in the other direction. I'm just scared of getting hurt again.

GIGI: That's very valid.

GOTTMIK: I think a lot of the competitive spirit in the trans community is brought upon ourselves, too. If someone's not trying to compete with us, we might still think that they are.

GIGI: Oh, that's an interesting outlook.

GOTTMIK: I'm just thinking about what my brain is constantly doing. It's like, *Oh, he's so buff. I need to be buffer,* or *His jawline is so masculine. I need filler.* And then suddenly, I have a long list of things to do: get filler, lift weights, eat healthy, whatever. I spiral. And the funny thing is the guys whose pictures I'm looking at are probably Facetuning.

GIGI:	Photoshopping.
GOTTMIK:	Right. And I know that, but somehow I still fall into the comparison trap. I'm like, *I need to be a masculine Greek god!*
GIGI:	You don't even want to be that though.
GOTTMIK:	I know. But somehow, I think I do sometimes. It feels almost involuntary. Obviously, I don't want to spiral, but my brain is like, *Sorry, it's happening.* And honestly, I think it's normal. I know that if I were a trans girl and I saw you, Gigi, I would be like, *Oh fuck, it's Barbie. I need to be Barbie!* And with trans guys who look like Ken, I think *I need to be Ken.* But the truth is that my aesthetic lies somewhere in between Barbie and Ken.
GIGI:	Envy is unhealthy.
GOTTMIK:	Yes.
GIGI:	But I fall into it, too. I see a nice pair of boobs, and I immediately want to know where I can get them.
GOTTMIK:	We also live in LA, where a lot of life for people is centered around looks.
GIGI:	The other thing to consider is that all trans guys and girls started in the same place, at the very beginning of a long transition, and we're all still in the process of transitioning, so it doesn't even make sense to compare.
GOTTMIK:	Right, and everyone's body reacts differently to different things. Some guys take testosterone and grow a beard fast. Other guys don't have that reaction. And that's not a thing you can change. That's just genetics. You can't control when your period's going to stop and when more hair is going to grow. I've been on testosterone for years, and I've only just started growing facial hair in the last few months. For a while,

I thought I was taking the wrong dose or something. I didn't understand that facial hair wasn't a given.

GIGI: In the last few years, I've arrived at a place of peace within myself. I really wish I could go back and tell the younger version of myself to be happier and not stress about the bullshit. As with everything else in life, there will be people ahead of you and people behind you. I wish I could tell younger me to really take it easy on herself. And I would say the same thing to any trans person who's just starting the process. Instead of comparing yourself to people on social media and feeling sad, focus on becoming happier within yourself.

GOTTMIK: A hundred percent.

GIGI: Ultimately, us feeling good about ourselves is what's going to further our trans community. We're already so far down the totem pole as it is, and it only drives us farther down when we're tearing each other apart.

GOTTMIK: Right. We need to stick together.

"As with everything else in life, there will be people ahead of you and people behind you."

Pageant Competitiveness

with **Sasha Colby**

PHOTO BY **PRESTON MENESES**

My first introduction to drag was through pageants, Miss Continental being the ultimate. Growing up in Hawaii, I would watch VHS tapes (yes, VHS) and find myself captivated by the glamour, talent, and extraordinary beauty of the contestants. I quickly learned that many of the competitors were trans, and that's when I got bit by the bug.

When I got to my first national pageant in 2005, I had just turned 21 and was in awe of everything in person. I mean this was the Academy Awards of drag. Audience members were so decked out in beautiful attire you couldn't tell who was in the pageant and who was a spectator.

The pageant world is a very unforgiving world. The whole point is to present the best version of yourself to then be judged mercilessly by not only the judges but by the audience. If the audience doesn't like you, you will know! If you do something amazing, you get roars and cheers; if you fumble, you get gasps and laughs. The drama of it all!

Speaking of drama, let me tell you about some crazy pageant stories that I've heard.

I've heard stories about a contestant going onstage for talent and by the time she comes back to her station to get into her gown, she discovers the gown has been cut up to the point that she would never be able to wear

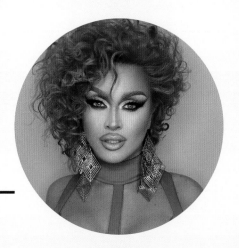

it. Now, we have security backstage and each contestant has a dresser who stays with your things to make sure no one tampers with it.

I've also heard of a lot of theft in pageants. Girls can't find their jewelry or hair, only to later find it in the alley dumpster. One story that always sticks out to me is one event in the '90s where Bob Mackie was judging Miss Continental and, during the gown competition, one contestant, who will remain unnamed, came out in a Bob Mackie gown. It was beautiful, and she looked exquisite. As soon as Mr. Mackie saw the gown he told the other judges that he only made two of that exact gown, one being in NYC for a magazine shoot and the other

having been stolen months ago from his store.

The queen in the gown was known for being a booster and always had labels on.

As soon as the contestant saw Mr. Mackie staring at her in shock on the judges panel, she finished modeling the gown, flitted off stage, and she, her entourage, and the gown had all vanished mid-pageant. She didn't stick around to experience any consequences, and the gown was never seen again. I often wonder if it's just sitting in a storage unit or closet somewhere unable to ever see the light of day.

Stand Together

with **Lina Bradford**

PHOTO BY **EMIL COHEN**

Trans people have been punchlines for comedians and ridiculed in mainstream media for years. So why do we continue to cut each other down within our own community? We're supposed to be this beautiful unified rainbow, and yet we are sometimes harsher with each other than the world is with us. If we want to make a difference for the next LGBTQ+ generation, then we need to be a better example. Let's show our younger siblings that we are more powerful when we stand together.

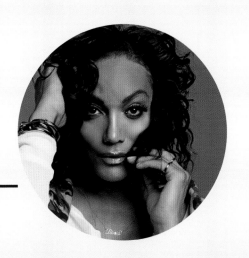

*"Why do we
continue to
cut each other
down within
our own
community?"*

Candis Cayne *on*

Competition Within the Community

PHOTO BY **NICK SPANOS**

Life in the trans community is exceptionally competitive. I think by nature a lot of our community feels a sense of competition in their career because, until recently, we didn't have a lot of options.

Back when I started my transition in 1995, there were three jobs that you could have as a trans person. You could be a showgirl, you could be a working girl, or you could be a makeup girl at MAC. Since then, our opportunities have widened and we are "allowed" in more spaces in society. But there is competition in all that we do.

I was the showgirl of the aforementioned job trifecta. I remember once when I was working at the clubs, I complimented a girl on how gorgeous she looked and she said, "Don't patronize me, Candis."

I was hurt by that for many years. Then, I got older and realized that the reason she'd said that to me was because something about me must have felt threatening to her. In other words, she thought I was the competition.

Now, instead of being angry, I'm sad for the loss of our friendship, but I'm also sad for her and how she lashed out.

Along with being a former showgirl, I did pageants. I also play sports and I'm an actress, so I know a

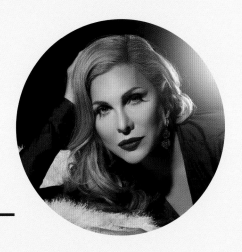

thing or two about being competitive. At some point along the way, I started to make a conscious effort to delineate between my competition in my career and competition with other trans girls.

I think competition between trans girls basically boils down to a scarcity mentality. For so long, there were no real opportunities, and by the time trans people started getting opportunities, this false idea that there wasn't enough for us all persisted.

"There's only one part, and there will never be another one!"

"There's only one job that will hire someone like us!"

"There's only one man who's interested, and that's not enough to go around!"

Statements like these are where our competitiveness lie. Honestly, I understand it. When you've lived in a world that is against you, and that hasn't offered you much opportunity, of course you're going to be scared and worried, and of course you'll do anything to get ahead.

My advice is to remember that the world is our oyster, we are unicorns, and whatever we set our minds to, we can achieve.

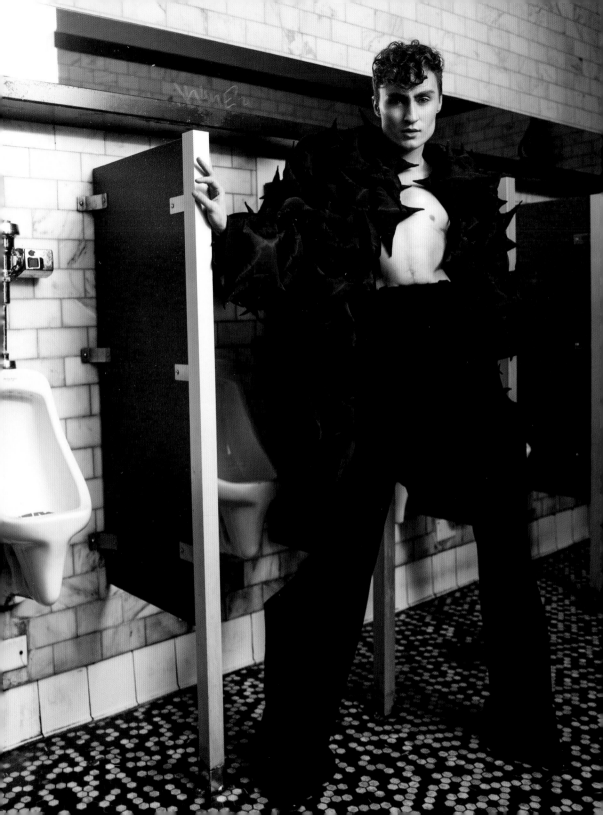

Public Restrooms

Public restrooms are notoriously triggering for trans people, so it's important to understand how to navigate them. As with so many other parts of the trans experience, there's no need to do it alone. Bring a buddy to the restrooms with you if you feel uncomfortable. If it's a cis friend who doesn't totally get it, clearly communicate your needs. Some allies need to be reminded to act as low-key guards. Public restrooms are a prime territory for shame and discomfort, so take extra good care of yourself. Most importantly, if you feel unsafe in any way, get out.

GIGI: The dreaded public restroom.

GOTTMIK: To me, it can be a very daunting thing for trans people. Whenever I see that gender sign on that door, I have to mentally prepare myself. I'm like, "Here we fucking go again." Before I go into a public restroom, I have to assess the situation. Here's a good example of how this can get tricky:

Recently, I went to an event where people knew who I was. They'd seen me on *Drag Race*. So, I didn't want to go to the girls' restroom, obviously, because I'm a man, but I didn't want to go to the guys' restroom either, because there's often only one stall and what if I had to stand in line and wait for it? Then everybody would know exactly why, which sounds ridiculous, but the thought of people thinking about my genitals in my presence gives me anxiety.

What did I do about this? I avoided the restroom situation completely.

Other situations can be a lot easier than this one, though. When I'm at the airport, which is usually full of the straightest men on the planet who aren't paying attention to me at all, I don't spiral about it. I just mind my business and go.

GIGI: Having to use the stall is a whole thing for trans guys.

GOTTMIK: I literally hate it. It's a very big trigger for me. I know some trans guys who could care less. It doesn't even cross their minds. Me, I need 10 minutes to recover after going to the restroom because I get so in my head about it. Whenever I have to use the stall, I convince myself that everyone else is thinking about why, even though that's probably not true. How upset I am depends on the location and time of day, really. If it's nighttime at a gay bar, it's not a huge deal. A lot of guys use the stalls. But in the daytime, at a nonqueer establishment, if I'm the only one waiting for a stall, then I start to get uneasy.

GIGI: I get that.

GOTTMIK: In my opinion, it's easier for trans guys, because men don't care as much about who's in their bathroom. I've never heard a guy say, "Get that girl out of the bathroom!" It's always the other way around.

GIGI: Totally.

GOTTMIK: Guys also have a bunch of different options. You can get stand-to-pee prosthetic packers, for example. Wearing one of those would probably solve a lot of my problems, but it would also create other problems. If I go out to a bar and I meet someone I want to hook up with, I don't want to have to say, "Oh, just a second," and then quickly take the prosthetic off. Talk about killing the moment.

GIGI: I feel like the restroom is a source of trauma for a lot of trans people. It's a dilemma that you have to constantly factor into everyday life. It's like, *Oh, let's go to a theme park for the day.* Then you get there and you're like, *Oh no, we're drinking fluids. I'm going to need to pee.* I know a lot of trans people who just don't go to the restroom for hours and hours.

Even before I came out as trans, I never felt like I belonged in the guys' restroom. It was weird for me that my peers would see me in there, so I would try to go only during class and never in between periods when the restroom was busy. I wanted to be the only one in the restroom, because keep in mind I was in full makeup at that time. I wasn't presenting as a boy, so the restroom was really triggering. If I couldn't sneak in there when it was empty, then I just wouldn't go.

GOTTMIK: Trans people holding it in for too long is such a thing.

GIGI: Here's my pro tip: use the buddy system. It might sound silly, but it makes all the difference in the world. Just grab a friend and say, "Come to the restroom." If they're cis and don't get it, you can quickly explain that you're gagging over the idea of having to go to the restroom alone and they need to come with you.

For a long time, I thought that going alone was better than explaining myself to my cis friends, who might not understand, but I don't think that anymore. What if something dangerous happened? You want a guard with you for safety reasons. Even someone standing outside the restroom and waiting for you is good. This is a much better option than getting stuck in an intimidating situation.

GOTTMIK: Buddy system is a hundred percent the vibe. I remember once, when I first started transitioning, I went to a gay bar in West Hollywood that weirdly had attendants in front of the restrooms. I went to the guys' restroom and was told, "You're not allowed in here," and then I went to the girls' restroom and was told the same thing.

GIGI: That's so awful.

GOTTMIK: I know. And this was a gay bar. And I had a buddy with me, who was also trans.

GIGI: That bar sounds so sketchy. I think in most situations, the buddy system works.

GOTTMIK: The other thing, which I barely want to talk about because it's such a trigger for me, is periods. Even growing up, I hated having my period and felt I needed to hide it from everyone. I was like, *People can't know this happens to me.* When I moved to LA and started transitioning, I could not handle buying tampons in front of people. I mean, I felt incapable of saying, "Hey, I need to stop at this store …" So I'd just have to figure something else out instead, which wasn't great. When I got on testosterone and my periods stopped, I was so relieved.

GIGI: I relate to that feeling of wanting to hide my body. Back in the day, I'd almost always take someone to the restroom with me and we'd go into the same stall, but I wouldn't let them watch me. Even now, when I take a girlfriend to the restroom, she knows to turn around, because I've said that so many times. "Turn around!" It's become an inside joke. I'd rather die than have anyone see me peeing or tucking, which seems similar to how you feel about your period.

"Here's my pro tip: use the buddy system. "

GOTTMIK: Totally.

GIGI: But I'll still bring friends to the restroom with me, for sure. Now it's easy because I've clearly communicated to them what I need so many times, so they're ready. They get it. And I feel so much safer. Honestly, tucking in a stall alone and then emerging from the restroom to face the other women in the bathroom is scary, and it can bring up shame.

GOTTMIK: I'm hoping that in the future, genitalia won't be widely associated with gender in the same way it is now.

GIGI: Right, like we shouldn't be calling them "feminine products." And it shouldn't be assumed that tucking is only for guys.

GOTTMIK: Yes. I was taught that only girls have their periods, which is not the case.

GIGI: There's so much stigma around genitalia.

GOTTMIK: Which is why restrooms are so triggering.

GIGI: The best thing you can do is get a confident, assertive trans or cis friend to be your low-key guard.

GOTTMIK: Do you think the restroom has gotten easier for you over time?

GIGI: Yes and no. It depends on where I am, how I'm presenting, and how sensitive I'm feeling. Sometimes, at the airport, I dress down. I don't wear a lash or makeup. I look less feminine, which makes me a little more uncomfortable with restrooms. But, what's changed is that I know how to handle my energy now. I hold my chin high up. I turn on the confidence. I've been trans for so long at this point that even at the straightest of straight spaces, I can turn it on. Still, some days are just harder than others. I feel rawer, and I'm just not in the mood to deal with restroom weirdness.

GOTTMIK: Right. Luckily I've never had anything terrible happen to me in a restroom, but that's definitely not the case for everyone.

GIGI: For a lot of trans people, the restroom is a lifelong battle.

GOTTMIK: I think asking for what you need is major. Once, I was on a tour bus in the UK. It was late at night and some of the guys needed to pee, so the driver just pulled over on the side of the road. I desperately had to pee, but there was no way I was going to squat out there. So I just held it. A better choice would have been to say to the driver, "Yo, I need a real restroom." I didn't do that because I was so in my head. And it was the same with periods. I think it's important to get comfortable talking about this stuff with your friends, even though I know that can feel so hard.

GIGI: The other thing is that you have to bring the right buddy to the restroom with you.

"I know how to handle my energy now. I hold my chin high up. I turn on the confidence."

GOTTMIK: Exactly. This is more advice to cis allies: don't point at the stall and make it a big deal about them needing the stall. Just let them go. Don't make it a thing. This sounds so obvious, but you don't know how many times guys have made a huge deal about getting a stall for me because I need it.

GIGI: Yes. I think all of this is good advice. The one thing I would add is about safety. If you get a weird vibe in a restroom, or if anybody says anything shady to you, get out immediately.

GOTTMIK: Especially if you're in a space that feels very nonqueer.

GIGI: Yes. Just leave. Your safety is number one.

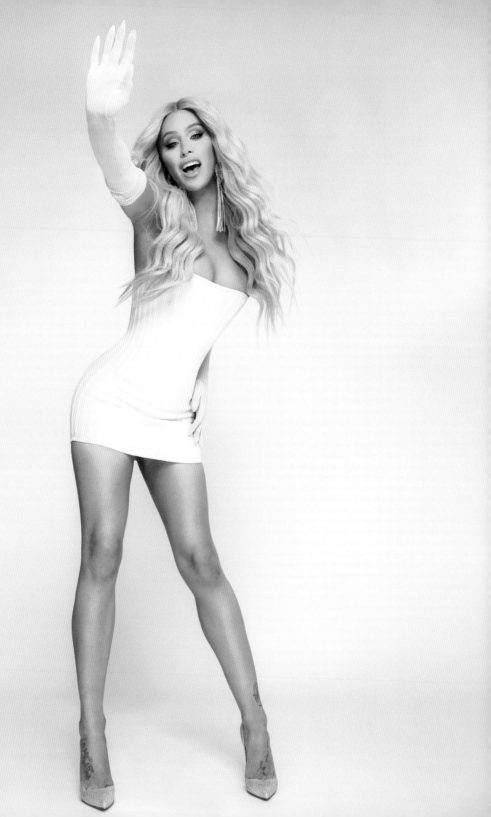

What to Do with Negativity

Dealing with negativity is part of every trans person's life, and it can appear in a variety of ways. Maybe somebody makes a mean comment online that gets under your skin, maybe somebody is rude or aggressive to you in person, or maybe you're the target of discrimination. It's unrealistic to think that you won't be affected by this type of stuff in your life, so the question is: what is the best way to deal with it?

GIGI: The biggest thing I've learned is that the hate that's coming at you has nothing to do with you. I've actually found that people who hate trans people often have queer preferences themselves. Everyone is in their own little world, thinking about themselves and their problems, and everything people say is a reflection of how they're feeling, not a reflection of who you are. It can be hard to remember this, so you have to train your mind. Maybe make your mantra, "This has nothing to do with me."

GOTTMIK: Exactly.

GIGI: That doesn't mean it's always easy, though, because it's not like we're robots. We're human. Still, even today, I can get a hundred positive comments and one negative comment and that one will haunt me.

GOTTMIK: I ignore online comments completely. I mean, *Drag Race* fandom is absolutely insane. When I got on the show, some people did not understand that I was trans. They'd call me a woman and accuse me of signing up just to get attention. I've received death threats. I don't delete mean comments, because I don't want to give anyone the satisfaction. I just leave them there and move on.

I've taken psych evaluations before going on TV shows, and a common question is how you deal with negative comments. I always say I ignore them. You have to remember that people are sitting at home hiding behind their screens, probably feeling bad about some part of their lives that has nothing to do with you. The internet makes it easy to be mean. In person, I rarely receive negative comments.

GIGI: Take the high road and don't engage is my advice. You're not going to change somebody's mind by chatting it out with them, and it's not your job to do that, so don't bother. I used to respond to mean comments, and often the person would end up apologizing. It's like they were just trying to get my attention. If what you want at the end of the day is peace of mind, then you can't be letting negativity from strangers who don't know you at all get under your skin.

GOTTMIK: Which is easier said than done sometimes.

GIGI: Right, because if you see a mean comment, it can hurt. It really depends what kind of mood you're in, too. If you're feeling insecure and sensitive already, it's harder, obviously. As a trans person in the spotlight, I just consider this to be part of the deal. If you're putting yourself out there, people are going to react to you, and not always in the ways that you want.

"If what you want at the end of the day is peace of mind, then you can't be letting negativity from strangers who don't know you at all get under your skin."

GOTTMIK: Yes. Another annoying thing that happens is when other trans people on the internet give you advice. They'll be like, "You need filler. You need lash extensions." Those type of comments really give me pause. I think, *Do I need these things?* As you said, Gigi, if you're putting yourself out there, then you need to get good at not letting other people affect you if you want to preserve your sanity. You can't get lost in the noise of what other people want for you. Your driving force should be your own desire.

GIGI: Ask yourself, "Is this me trying to get validation? Or is this me doing this for me?"

GOTTMIK: No need to let people give you complexes.

GIGI: Speaking of which, I have a trans girlfriend who was telling me that her trans girlfriend kept asking her about FFS. "When are you getting it? When are you getting it?" Apparently, she just would not stop bringing it up. She wanted them to book FFS appointments together and make it a joint thing. My friend, after checking in with herself, realized that she never wanted FFS. She's happy with her face as it is. It works for her. But, she got confused when her friend kept bringing it up. And the friend probably thought she was being helpful, too. It's just that unsolicited advice is often not useful.

GOTTMIK: It's a vulnerable position to be in when you're transitioning, which means that people giving you bad advice can be dangerous. When you're new to the landscape, you're not sure what's right for you yet and it's easy to get lost. At the start of my drag career, when I was painting my face white all the time because it's ambiguous, people kept telling me to stop. They were like, "Do a skin tone!" And I did, eventually, but not until I was ready.

What's hard is when you're listening to people but you're not even totally aware that you're listening. It's that subtle influence that can be tricky. Sometimes, things are moving so fast that it takes me a minute to notice that my style has shifted in a way that mirrors somebody else's but that isn't ultimately me. It's so easy to follow trends when that's what everyone seems to like, but staying true to who I am as an artist and a person is the only way to grow.

GIGI: Same. And I think being in the public eye forces you to define yourself.

GOTTMIK: The number one question I get is, "What advice would you give to a drag queen who wants to stand out?" And my answer is always that you need to lean in to whatever makes you unique. The second you start trying to follow trends, it's game over. What people connect to is literally *you* and no one else. You don't have to do what other people are doing. You can be the taste maker. Of course, some people aren't going to like it.

GIGI: Everybody can't like everything.

GOTTMIK: Right.

GIGI: So the best thing to do is try and let the negativity roll right off you.

Know Your Truth

with **Schuyler Bailar**

PHOTO BY **VIOLETTA MARKELOU**

The first day I accepted that I was transgender, I spent hours in tears, sobbing and panicking. I was afraid of what I expected was to come—the impending discrimination, pain, arguments, loss, and grief were all consuming. That day, I felt more alone and lost than ever before. As a recruited women's collegiate athlete, I was certain my transness was the worst thing I could ever discover about myself. What if I lose everything?

That day was more than eight years ago now. All that I expected did happen—I cannot count the number of death threats or the hateful messages I've received, the nights I've stayed awake anxious and in pain from the transphobia in my personal world, and the seemingly never-ending legislative attacks launched against us. Despite any setbacks, I am also certain that being trans is, unequivocally, magic. My transness has afforded me a perspective that most cisgender people can never access. I have walked through the world perceived as a myriad of identities, and what a wonderful experience it is to hold all this conflicting, beautiful nuance along the journey of finding myself and my happiness.

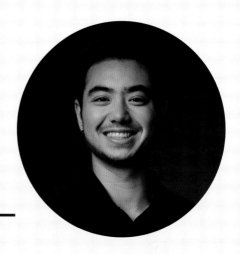

I often tell my mother that the womanhood she taught me has made me the man I am today. I did not jump out of the box of womanhood to be shoved into someone else's box of manhood; and so, I hold my womanhood close. It has informed so much of how I walk through the world, how I welcome my femininity, and how I find my gentle masculinity in a culture too often demanding toxicity and stoicism.

As we weather more anti-trans legislation and violence than ever before, it is all the more important to remember the power of our identities and our agency in them. No matter how many laws they pass or how many of our rights they attempt to deny, they can never take away our identities. That is, I will always be transgender—in every state, under any law, in any bathroom or doctor's office, on the field or in the pool, in any sport I play...No lawmaker can take this identity from me. No governor can erase my knowledge of myself. I will always know my own truth. And that is perhaps one of the most powerful proofs of resilience our community will never lose.

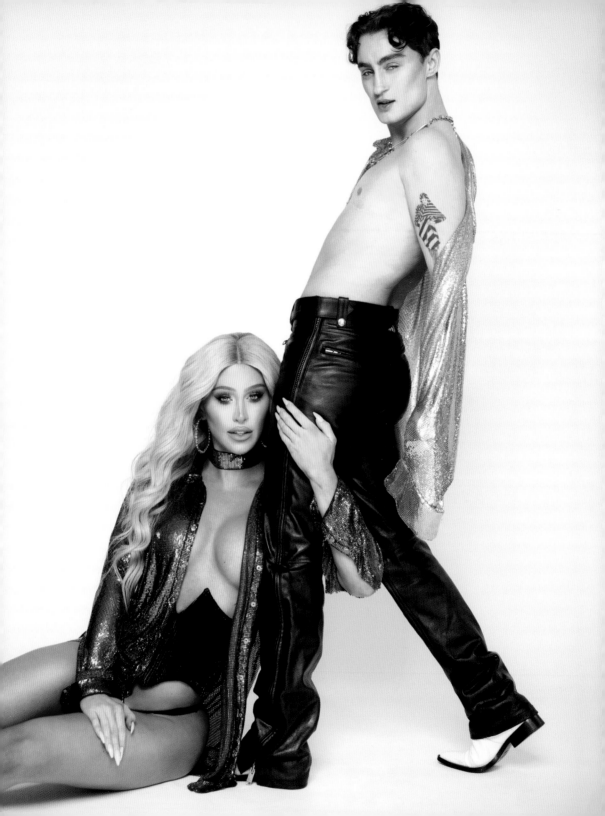

Dating

Dating is a huge subject for many people, and for trans people, it's even bigger and more complex. When you transition, you often get curious about your body in a new way, which can lead to an exploratory period. This can often be a healthy and wonderful time to get to know yourself on a deeper level. But, as a newbie, you're in a vulnerable position, possibly prone to second-guessing yourself, and this type of mentality can be slightly dangerous when you're getting involved with people who don't want the best for you.

Another issue that often comes up for trans people is disclosure. When should you divulge to a prospective lover that you're trans? Are you lying by not telling them? And after you do tell them, how can you make sure you're safe if you get a negative reaction?

As trans people go along, many of them change their views about their sexuality, which obviously impacts who they date. We both came out as pan somewhere along the way. There are so many misconceptions when it comes to sexuality and gender in the romantic sphere, and trans people often get a lot of questions that straight people definitely don't, such as, "Do you have a vagina or a penis?"

What's very uncommon in the trans community is marriage. Even though it's finally legal in the United States, many trans people aren't doing it. Why is that? We'll try to answer that question in this section, as well as get into all the other complexities of dating as a trans person.

GIGI: When I ask myself what it's been like to date as a transgender woman, the first word that comes to mind is *scary.* It felt so stressful because I wasn't sure when to divulge that I was trans. I wanted to be honest, but it's also such an awkward thing to say when you first meet someone and you don't even know what kind of relationship you're going to have with them yet. Also, what if they already know? I would go out to a club and meet someone and think, *Am I lying by not telling this person I'm trans right now, or is it none of their business?*

GOTTMIK: Waiting for the reveal moment.

GIGI: Right. And sometimes, when they found out, they'd say something that would give me the ick. I'd feel fetishized, which I hate. When you become a fetish, it's like you're no longer a real person. Every time that happened, I would immediately lose respect for the guy. When I first moved to LA, it was a lot of dating and a lot of nothingness. I just felt so lonely. Was every guy going to fetishize me? Would I always be made to feel horrible? I started getting worried that it would never change.

GOTTMIK: I think with dating in general, you're not going to get anywhere unless you feel comfortable with yourself. Being trans is that times a million. If you don't really know who you are yet, or you're trying to figure it out, trying to find that through someone else, especially people who are going to fetishize you, is going to be a disaster. I felt fetishized, too, when I first started to transition. So, I took a break from hooking up with people. I decided I wasn't going to let people into my life in an intimate way until I'd created some intimacy with myself.

Recently, I've gotten back into dating. I'm mostly into gay guys, and since most gay guys have seen *Drag Race*, I'm usually not left wondering if they know I'm trans or not. But there have been times when the topic of the show hasn't come up, and I'm not sure how the guy is perceiving me. What I do then is say, "Hey, have you seen *Drag Race?*" This a way for me to see if they know my story or not.

On the apps, I just write that I'm trans in my bio. With certain guys, I double check just to make sure. "You know I'm trans, right?" I'll say something like that. And it's really interesting. A lot of guys get aggressive. Like, "Yeah, I can fucking read." Or they'll shut down and not want to talk about it. I think they must feel ashamed.

GIGI: Bringing it up is the worst, and reactions are often the worst, too. I've had guys say to me, "Oh, I don't mind dick." Which just made me feel so bad. And then, too, there's the anxiety leading up to the moment of the reveal. You're sitting there trying to phrase it in your head. "I wasn't born a girl …" So awkward.

When I was younger, I knew who I was, but I didn't know who I was when it came to romance. I'd only been in one relationship before transitioning. What I learned is that I couldn't count on outside sources to give me validation. Searching for that from a man is just a waste of time. It has to come from within you.

GOTTMIK: People say the craziest things.

GIGI: Yes, and trans people are oversexualized. I can't tell you how many times I've been asked, "Do you have a penis or a vagina?" As if it's anyone's business.

GOTTMIK: That question is not okay.

GIGI: No, it's not. But there's the other problem of not breaching the topic at all, because then you're thinking, *What do they know? What are they thinking?* Trans dating is regular dating, but on crack. Which is why I think a lot of trans people feel lonely.

GOTTMIK: Yes.

GIGI: They either don't date at all, because it's so depressing to be made to feel fetishized, or they go for it, and because striking gold is so rare, a lot of them end up settling for someone who's mediocre but really accepting.

GOTTMIK: Every day in my DMs: Do you have a penis or a vagina?

GIGI: Even now that I'm married, people will still ask me that.

GOTTMIK: And then the sexualized comments that follow can be even worse. "Oh, I want to eat you out."

GIGI: Hello, we're real humans. If you're on the apps, I think it's a good idea to divulge your transness in your bio.

GOTTMIK: And then you can avoid the awkwardness of having to say it out loud.

GIGI: It's also just a safety issue. You don't want to go out with somebody who doesn't know and then have them react in a violent way.

GOTTMIK: Right. And when I meet people out in real life, I like to let them know early. If they react in a weird way, I move on.

GIGI: Safety first.

GOTTMIK: Recently, I got into a situation that kind of made me feel like a hypocrite. I was hooking up with this trans girl, who I guess I assumed hadn't had bottom surgery, which turned out to be wrong. I encountered a full-on vagina, which was not what I expected. It had been a really long time since I'd hooked up with a girl, so I was unprepared. After a moment of shock, I quickly realized that I hate it when people judge other people according to their genitalia, and that's exactly what I was doing. Anyway, then I got into it and it was fun.

GIGI: Wait, I love that.

GOTTMIK: Isn't that crazy? I can't believe I assumed I knew what her genitalia would be. So gross of me.

GIGI: The other thing about the apps is that you have to be wary of the guys with bad intentions who go on there hunting for trans people.

GOTTMIK: Yes. I have a friend who went to meet a guy from an app, and the guy showed up with a friend. She ended up getting into their car, and they beat her up.

GIGI: That's fucked.

GOTTMIK: And they robbed her at gunpoint.

GIGI: I'd be traumatized if that happened to me.

GOTTMIK: I know. And I have another friend who just got beat up in a similar situation. It's crazy. She blasted it online, but justice has not been served.

GIGI: I think a lot of trans girls want to stay silent when shady stuff happens. They just kind of sweep it under the rug. I have found myself doing that, honestly, about little things. It rarely happens, but it's a wake-up call to me every time it does. We all need to be louder.

GOTTMIK: I'm extra careful dating on the apps. I haven't done it a lot, but when I do, I make sure I'm safe. I definitely won't go meet anyone alone. I'll say, "Me and my friends are out. Come meet us."

GIGI: Such a good one.

GOTTMIK: Then when they show up you catch their vibe, but there's a lot less pressure.

GIGI: What about asking to FaceTime? I feel like if they say no, that's a red flag. Meeting people out is the best, though.

GOTTMIK: You can tell a lot by the way somebody's chatting with you, too. If it seems creepy, get out.

GIGI: I think trans people sometimes like to think that they're the same as cis people when it comes to dating, but the truth is that we are extremely special and we need to be a little bit more careful. I know that if I were a 21-year-old on the apps, newly transitioning and curious, I'd read that and be like, "Sure, whatever." But this is actually monumentally important. Be careful.

GOTTMIK: So careful.

GIGI: Be on your toes.

GOTTMIK: We need to talk about how we've both become pan. I feel that a change in sexual identity is highly related to the dating and love category.

GIGI: Yes. Learning more about myself over the years is what allowed me to change. Now, I fully identify as pan, but a few years ago, I didn't even know what that was. It's inevitable that as you grow, your ideas about yourself and who you're attracted to are going to change.

As I mentioned before, my dad's always calling me asking me when I'm getting bottom surgery. It's so funny. I'm like, "Dad! We were talking about fucking lunch plans! I'll let you know." For a very long time, I wasn't sure that I wanted bottom surgery. I was thriving without it. And then when I met Nats, he identified as a woman, which was new. I'd made out with girls at the club, but that was it. I'd only dated guys. But the more I leaned in to my relationship with Nats, the more I liked it. After a while, it hit me: *Oh, I'm gay again!* Actually, coming out as gay showed me how much more comfortable I'd become with myself compared to the first two times I'd come out—as a gay man and then as a trans woman.

GOTTMIK: And now Nats has come out as trans.

GIGI: And I'm pan. I have to say, I do love a label! I mean, obviously. I've come out four times. But more seriously, Nats has taught me that I can fall in love with anyone. It's not contingent on gender. Figuring this out about myself is part of my evolution and part of my growth, I feel. Before, I was blocking myself off from love, partly because of my own insecurities.

GOTTMIK: I think one thing that can happen when a trans person's sexuality changes over time is that people then assume their gender should be negated. People often ask me why I would transition to being a guy if I was just going to date guys. Gender and sexuality are completely different, as we said before.

GIGI: Yes.

GOTTMIK: I feel like my being pan speaks to my growth, too, and to my openness. I feel so much better now that I've decided that genitalia isn't everything.

GIGI: Right. It's limiting. If I didn't open it up, I wouldn't be married right now.

GOTTMIK: Let's hear the story of how you fell for him … when he was still living as a female.

GIGI: Nats's brother, who I'd been friends with for a while, introduced us. And, I don't know, from the very beginning, it just felt like we had really good vibes. It was strange for me, and totally unexpected. I was like, *What is happening right now? Why am I into this?* I had never thought I might be into women. It just wasn't even a question in my mind. And then, suddenly, it was happening. And the only reason I was open to it was because I felt really good within myself. I needed validation from the outside, and I was more in touch with what I was actually feeling.

Later, when Nats transitioned, it made sense to me. He'd always been very masculine, and people would often misgender him out in public. I didn't think very much of it. But when he was like, "I think I want to transition. I think I want top surgery," I got into it fast. I was like, "You don't have to say anything else. I'm pro top surgery. I'm pro trans. Let's do this." I was so in love with him already. I would have been smitten with him in any form.

GOTTMIK: Did you always want to get married?

GIGI: I mean, I wasn't that little kid who always thought about her wedding day and what she was going to wear. I was never that deep into it, but I knew that I did want kids and a partner. In the distance, I always imagined a husband, a house, pets, and kids. But in reality, I didn't think it was necessarily in the cards, because I spent a lot of years being promiscuous and getting bored of people fast. I wasn't the type to fall in love easily, or for long. I'd date someone for a month and then realize I couldn't stand them. The longest relationship I was in pre-Nats was two years, but I was cheating constantly. It wasn't love. I can see that now. It was just stupid.

So, even though I thought it would be nice to get married, I also thought I'd never be that lucky. Maybe I felt unlovable to a certain degree. Maybe I thought I didn't deserve to be loved so fully. They say it finds you when you're not looking for it, and that certainly was the case with me. I wasn't looking for Nats at all.

GOTTMIK: I think we should talk about marriage when it comes to the trans community.

GIGI: Totally.

GOTTMIK: I watch this show *Pose,* and in one episode, a trans girl gets married. She and all her friends are celebrating together, and she decides to make it everyone's wedding day, since nobody else in the group is married.

GIGI: That's so chill.

GOTTMIK: I was sobbing.

GIGI: That's cute.

GOTTMIK:	So many trans people, and gay people, think they can never get married.
GIGI:	Do you want to get married?
GOTTMIK:	Only if we can have separate bedrooms.
GIGI:	That's hilarious.
GOTTMIK:	But the real answer is maybe, just not yet.
GIGI:	I don't think I know many other trans people who are married. Do you?
GOTTMIK:	Ummm … no. Isn't that weird? I'm sure there are lots of married trans people out there—we just don't know them.
GIGI:	During my wedding, I was so immersed in my fairytale that I wasn't even thinking about what a big deal it was. Then, later, I was like, *Whoa.* I remember my friend said, "Bitch, trans people don't get married. Trans people are sex workers."
GOTTMIK:	It's everything to your fans, and for the community in general.

"In the distance, I always imagined a husband, a house, pets, and kids."

GIGI: Yeah, we're really loud about our relationship. And we get a lot of nice messages about how our marriage makes people feel hopeful. I really never thought it would happen to me.

GOTTMIK: I almost feel like I've convinced myself that I don't need marriage, and I wonder how much that has to do with there being so few precedents in my life.

GIGI: I think it's good not to dwell on what you're potentially missing. Like I said, I met Nats when I wasn't looking for anyone. If you spend your time putting pressure on finding a relationship or getting married, it will consume you, and you'll just be upset waiting for it to happen. It's detrimental to lose sleep over something you have no control over. I think trusting fate is probably a better way to go. Relationship or not, you want to be thriving. Get busy. Focus on the things you love. And then if the right person comes along, great. They're adding to the equation, but you don't need them to survive.

GOTTMIK: I feel like I'm in a moment of focusing on myself right now. I've spent all this time trying to build a career, and it's finally happening. There are also surgeries I want, which I know are going to make me feel even more aligned with how I want to look. I know I can be a perfectionist, though, and I know thinking I need to be perfect in order to meet someone isn't the right headspace to be in, because there will always be something to tweak.

GIGI: Totally.

GOTTMIK: Eventually, I'll look for a long-term relationship, I think. Right now, I'm loving the chaotic, fast-paced energy of my life. I can't imagine needing to stay in the same city for too long or needing to text somebody back. Like, "Leave me alone, I'm partying!"

GIGI: Hilarious.

GOTTMIK: We need to go back to the validation thing for a second, because I think that applies to all types of relationships. Long-term, short-term, one-night stands. I have a lot of trans girlfriends who find themselves drawn into sexual situations that I don't think are healthy. They'll be like, "I'm going to this orgy," and I get worried that they're allowing themselves to be treated like little sex objects. When you're out and drinking, it's easy to think that bad decisions aren't that bad, but when you wake up sober, it's a different experience. I think it's bad for your soul to be used sexually, or in any way.

GIGI: Right. I think in the beginning, it can feel good to experiment. But definitely making choices when you're drunk is not the best.

GOTTMIK: Yeah, it's all in the spirit of fun, but then the truth is that it's dark. When you're just starting to transition, there's so much to navigate, and it can be really hard to know what's best for you. Also, as we said before, it's a vulnerable time, and sex is a vulnerable act. I wish all my trans girlfriends would treat themselves like the precious beings they are.

GIGI: I think it's about knowing your value. But if you feel unlovable, then it's natural in a way to seek out situations that reinforce that.

GOTTMIK: Yes.

GIGI: Instead of us teaching people how to treat us, we sometimes let other people teach us how we're going to be treated.

GOTTMIK: I guess if it's fun, keep doing it. Just make sure you're asking yourself if you're happy.

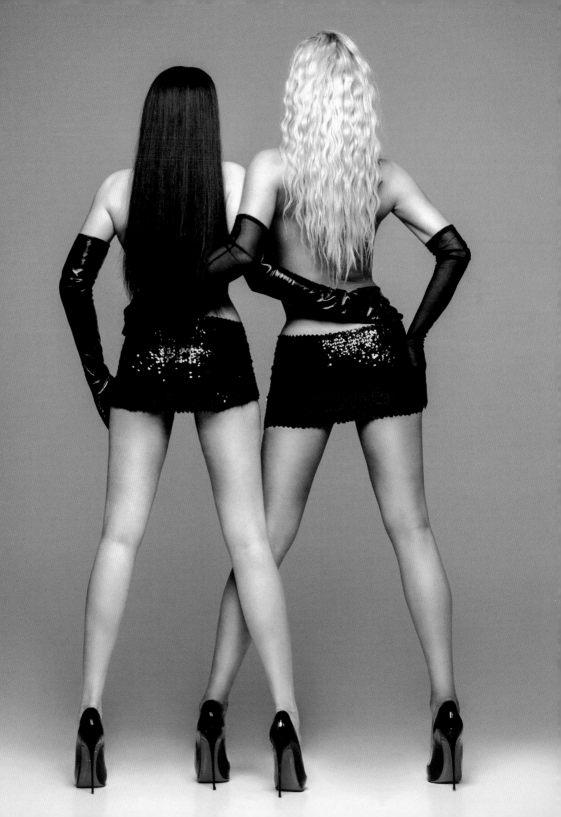

Advocating for Yourself

A lot of trans people struggle with their own worthiness. The less worthy we feel, the less we advocate for ourselves. In this section, we're going to tell you a little bit about how we've learned to protect ourselves and make smart decisions in our careers. We expect that some of the specific info about the entertainment industry will be totally unrelatable for many of you, but the accompanying emotions are universal and apply especially to any entrepreneurial type who's trying to carve a path for themselves. We're also going to touch upon tokenism in this section, which is, unfortunately, somewhat common in "woke" circles.

GOTTMIK: 2021 was supposed to be the best year of my life. After *Drag Race,* I signed with a new management company. They booked me for all these appearances around the world, and suddenly, I was on a plane every other day, arriving in a new city. It all happened so fast, and I was making so much money, more money than I'd ever made before. I loved it. I thrived on the chaos—even though at times, it was a little too chaotic. I'd be given a schedule at the last minute and have to go right to the airport and get on another plane. I never knew in advance which venue had booked me or what my rate was. I was just going, going, going.

Then, in the winter, everything slowed down. December and January are notoriously slow for events. In that time, I was able to take a step back and remember the real goals I had before the chaos. I was like, *Wait, what happened to the makeup line I wanted to start? What about the acting I want to do? And the singing?* I realized that all I'd been doing was making money for this management company. What did I have to show for the last year? Not that much. Anyway, it was an aha moment. I was like, *I need to take control of my career!*

GIGI: And not become another stereotypical drag queen.

GOTTMIK: Yes, because when I looked back at the year, it made me sad. Yes, I'd made money, but I hadn't had any time to myself and I hadn't produced any tangible art. After the fun wore off, I felt empty. I was just chasing this shiny thing.

Here's what ended up happening: I left the management company. And it got really dramatic really fast. They kicked me off the tour, wired me some money, and basically said, "Good luck, babe." The circumstances of the ending were unfortunate, but ultimately it was an important moment for me. I felt like by leaving, I was advocating for the career I wanted.

GIGI: Good for you.

GOTTMIK: Thank you. I learned later that we were only being paid a small
            fraction of what they were charging the venues, and that the
            management company was saying no to jobs on my behalf without
            checking with me in order to keep me on tour.

GIGI: Gross.

GOTTMIK: Right. So, I'd make them more money. They didn't care about my
            career goals or me as a person. They just wanted money.

GIGI: As you know, I've had a bad experience with this company, too.

GOTTMIK: People are shady. This is an exciting moment for drag queens in the
            media, and they take advantage of it. Things are changing drastically
            for us. Up until now, drag queens didn't go to fashion week, let alone
            be in Versace campaigns! We're finally moving into the mainstream.

GIGI: And being used like circus animals by some people.

GOTTMIK: Right.

GIGI: *Drag Race* is such an amazing show, because it's opened doors for drag
            queens in a major way. All this press and all these events are so
            empowering to the community—but then there's this greedy dark side,
            which I guess is what happens when there's a lot of money at stake.

GOTTMIK: *Drag Race* as a show has almost single-handedly changed the world of
            drag. The first few seasons reflect how drag used to be viewed—as an
            underground, punk rock form of self-expression. Back then, to stand
            out as a contestant, you had to be an icon. Drag queens were unique.
            Each had her own flavor. Early on in the show, you can see that each
            character is so different. Now drag is so accessible. Which is amazing
            on many levels. We want to be seen. But the impact on drag as a form
            of art has been negative in some ways. Everybody uses the same tricks
            now, and everybody kind of looks the same. That's not great, because

where's the creativity? When things get popular, they often get homogenous, which sucks.

GIGI: Totally.

GOTTMIK: The other big impact of us becoming mainstream is that everyone is vying for the same big jobs. Who's going to be the first drag queen to get a Coca-Cola commercial, for example? Who's going to be the first to walk in a Chanel show?

GIGI: I feel that we're getting back into the subject of competition.

GOTTMIK: Exactly. It's drag queens trying to tear other drag queens down.

GIGI: I believe that there's enough pie for everyone. Everyone in the queer community needs to remember that.

GOTTMIK: A hundred percent. Early on in my *Drag Race* season, a castmate of mine got a major campaign, and I felt so envious at first. I was like, *Wait, where's mine?* It took me a second to remember that every time someone in the queer community books a big job like that, it's a win for the whole community. We are all pushing the conversation forward.

GIGI: We're fighting the same fight.

GOTTMIK: And we're all different. The job that was right for my castmate isn't the right job for me, but the next job might be. Brands are looking for specific things, and sometimes you're just not the thing they're looking for.

GIGI: It's not even personal.

GOTTMIK: So, you can't even really take it as a rejection.

GIGI: One billion percent. Nobody is taking your slice of pie, because it wasn't yours to begin with.

GOTTMIK: What's so great is that after I left that management company, all of these opportunities came in. I'm now getting paid full rates and working with people who are supportive. It took a lot of work to rebuild my team, but it was so worth it.

GIGI: Absolutely.

GOTTMIK: I'm so happy.

GIGI: What's going on with your makeup line now?

GOTTMIK: The short version is that it's slowly coming together. Once you have a platform, there's some pressure to rush through this type of stuff. Like, "Who cares how good it is. They'll buy it." But I'm taking my time.

GIGI: I always forget you have a degree in product development.

GOTTMIK: I know. I'm really excited about it. I have some cool ideas.

GIGI: I think what every queer entrepreneurial soul needs to focus on is being themselves. Everything good stems from that.

GOTTMIK: And you have to trust your intuition. There were so many red flags with this management company that I ignored. I got so caught up in the money and the excitement that I forgot to ask myself what I really wanted to be doing with my time.

GIGI: I feel like you're really moving forward in your career now, and that it's only happening because you're doing exactly what you want.

GOTTMIK: Thank you. Should we talk about how you learned to advocate for yourself in your career?

GIGI: Sure. I'll start at the beginning for context. So, our manager Scott actually hit me up in Toronto just as I was starting to form a presence on social media. He was like, "Hey, I have this idea for a reality show …" Basically, it was a Canadian version of *The Hills*, which was popular at the time. I ended up meeting Scott at his apartment in Toronto. I guess I'd maybe expected him to be some 40-year-old guy, but it turned out he was a college student at Ryerson University, and only 2 years older than me.

GOTTMIK: So funny.

GIGI: I know. He was like, "Want to do this reality show and I'll manage you?" Obviously, I said yes. And after the show, all these opportunities started pouring in. It was one thing after another. Eventually, Scott started his company and now he's in LA.

GOTTMIK: You got lucky with him. He's so supportive and amazing and sweet.

GIGI: I know. He's Canadian. Which makes the story extra crazy. Most Canadians aren't thinking about how to create reality shows and manage talent … especially when they're in college.

GOTTMIK: It's insane.

GIGI: We were just kids when we met.

GOTTMIK: Iconic.

GIGI: Yes, but I've still totally had shady people advocating for me.

GOTTMIK: Please do tell.

GIGI: Many years ago, I did this job with Kylie Jenner. It was easy and fun, and the money was good. But I'd hired this new PR agency, and basically their way of promoting the collab was to say that Kylie and I were best friends. I was still new to LA, and I thought, *Is this what publicity is here?* I felt very uncomfortable. So, I ended up firing that agency.

GOTTMIK: You did a little pivot.

GIGI: With Scott by my side, yeah.

GOTTMIK: Any other moments in your career when you've felt taken advantage
           of?

GIGI: I mean, I've definitely felt like the token trans girl more than once. I've
           been hired with a "let's check the trans box" mentality. For a long time,
           I just felt so honored to be welcomed into any room. Whatever the job
           was, I'd be like, "Yes!" It was often lost on me when I was younger that I
           was the token trans girl on a job or at an event. A friend would say
           something like, "Were there any other trans girls at that event?" And I
           would be like, "Oh, I guess I was the only one." It's disappointing to
           realize that the people aren't always driven by good morals.

GOTTMIK: I think it can be complicated, though, because even though being
           hired to check a box isn't ideal, any visibility is a good thing for the
           community.

GIGI: Totally. For me now, it depends on what the brand is and how much
           reach it has. If Google wants to hire me as their token trans girl, then
           great.

GOTTMIK: Right, and the values of the company matter. If they're donating to the
           right causes, and they have a history of celebrating Pride and being in
           the community in some sort of way, then I'd be happy to check a box
           for them. But being the token trans angel for a random brand that's
           never done anything for queer people and now only cares because it's
           cool? That's so not my vibe.

GIGI: It's like putting the rainbow in the window for Pride month because
           you feel like you're lame otherwise.

GOTTMIK: I need to talk about the big retailer that's selling drag merch that
           features me.

GIGI: Let's talk about it.

GOTTMIK: Okay, so this retailer does a ton to showcase the queer community in its stores. It sells massive amounts of merch during Pride. Is this retailer promoting queer life the rest of the year? Not as heavily, it seems, which kind of makes it seem like they're just cashing in on Pride month. Then again, because they're pushing such an astounding amount of merch, it's kind of forgivable.

GIGI: And they're huge.

GOTTMIK: Yeah, and it's so cool to see drag queen merch there. If I was a high schooler and I saw that, I would feel hope.

GIGI: Exactly.

GOTTMIK: That's a happy story for me. But I have sad ones for sure. During Pride, a lot of questionable motives get highlighted, I feel.

GIGI: Yes.

GOTTMIK: I talk a lot about these companies that feel pressured to participate but that don't really care about queer people. Once, I was doing a Pride event with a bunch of other people. The company sent me a flyer and asked me to promote it on my social media. The uncool part was that my name was literally at the very bottom of the flyer and almost nobody else listed was even queer. And all of them had fewer followers than I do. Which made me feel like I'd definitely been hired to check a box, and possibly also to promote the event.

GIGI: Gross.

GOTTMIK: Here's another example of this: There's a designer who hires all these drag queens and amazing queer artists for their Pride campaigns. And then, at the fashion show, they're all sitting in the second row. It's the same as being on the bottom of the flyer. Why not put us somewhere that is visible? I think it's often because the people who are chosen to sit in the front row are considered to be more palatable. And we, meanwhile, are queer bait.

GIGI: Pride month queer bait.

GOTTMIK: The worst is when you find out that a company that appears to be supportive during Pride month is actually donating to anti-gay organizations.

GIGI: Honestly, I really only realized that companies queer bait within the past couple years. I always just thought that it was cute how everyone throws up a flag during Pride month. But now I think it's so fucked up that these companies aren't behind the community the rest of the year. I love that people are talking about this now, though. I think it's progress for sure.

GOTTMIK: Total progress, but it still sucks that as a trans person, you're used as a puppet and sometimes discriminated against.

GIGI: I agree.

GOTTMIK: For a while, I was working as a makeup artist for this brand. I was freelance, but I basically worked for them every day. They gave me VIP passes to Coachella and invited me to stay in a house, which they invited very few artists to. Then I took a break to get top surgery. I came back a little bit too early, and it was very hard to work. I didn't do a bad job. I was just slower. And after that day, I was never asked to do makeup there again.

For a long time, I thought it was because I was slow or that I hadn't done the makeup in the way that they wanted. But then, much later, I told a friend about it and he said, "I think you got discriminated against. Why would they have randomly fired you?" So, that was a moment of reckoning for me. Because when my friend said that, I thought he was probably correct.

GIGI: I think it's so important that people know what their rights are, especially at work. If you feel like something is off, trust that feeling.

GOTTMIK: Yeah, I think it's always a good idea, too, to find some allies at work. A lot of the time, you can't see that something is off in the moment, so it's helpful when somebody else can point it out.

GIGI: Yes to allies in the workplace. Back when I was a boy in Canada wearing makeup, I got a job at this clothing store. I noticed that I was getting all these mean looks from customers who walked in. It was horrible. So, I made it a point to make friends with my coworker, who was also my boss, because I didn't want to feel alienated and alone at work. It turned out that she was into makeup, so we ended up forming a cute little bond.

GOTTMIK: Love it.

GIGI: I think sexual harassment in the workplace is another big one for trans women. Because we're frequently oversexualized, and because we tend to want to sweep shady behavior under the rug. I think I've probably been harassed and not even realized it until later.

GOTTMIK: It's amazing how often something shady happens and we don't realize it until way later, because we're so busy pretending like we're fine.

GIGI: In your gut, you always know when you're not fine.

GOTTMIK: A hundred percent.

GIGI: And that's the first step to advocating for yourself. First, you have to identify what's wrong, and then you have to identify what you want. The more worthy you feel, the more you will ask for, because you'll know that you deserve it. I think that in order to advocate for ourselves at work and in life, we need to know our worth. For me, my feelings of worthiness have grown over time. I wouldn't accept a lot of behavior now that I would have accepted in the beginning.

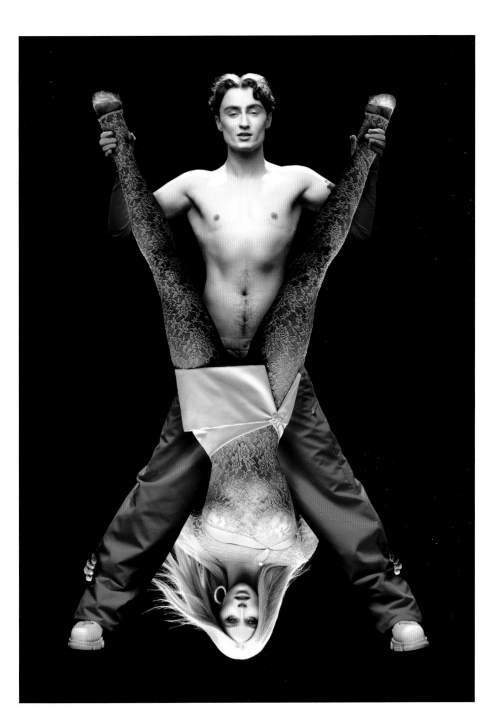

Stay
Present

with Laith Ashley

PHOTO BY **MARTIN SALGO**

I've been on testosterone for nine years, a milestone I'm so proud to have reached. It feels as though my journey began both so long ago and just yesterday. Many young guys reach out to me on social media, looking for answers to how I came up with my fitness routine, how I built my physique, and how taking testosterone changed me. My response is always "It takes time."

Early in my journey, I had most of the same questions these guys have—the same fears, too. But the early uncertainty is just one small blip on the overall path to becoming who you truly are.

Identifying as someone who is and appears more masculine, I wanted to be this perfect idea of the man in my head. I wanted the affirmation. Even before taking testosterone, I dressed and wore my hair in a more masculine fashion. After I started taking testosterone, feeling more confident in my skin, and witnessing the changes I wanted to see with my body, I actually

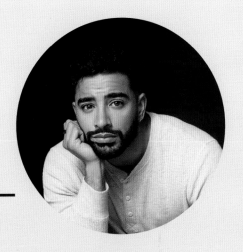

started stepping into my femininity a lot more. I feel like I'm much more feminine now than I was prior to transitioning!

At the end of the day, we're all in the gender expression community, none of us being completely male or female in a traditional sense. As a queer person, especially, I'm so honored to be a part of this community. I'm happy that I got to experience my life pre-transition, and that I now get to experience it in a more authentic way. I put in the work to build this body because it's what I like and what makes me feel good. I know that anybody in the modeling industry can relate to the pressure of maintaining their looks, but we also need to remember to be kind to ourselves. Remember that no one is perfect. Remember that the closer we get to an idea of perfection in our heads, the further we stray from it. It's moments like these that remind me I need to stay present, because that's what's most important in this life.

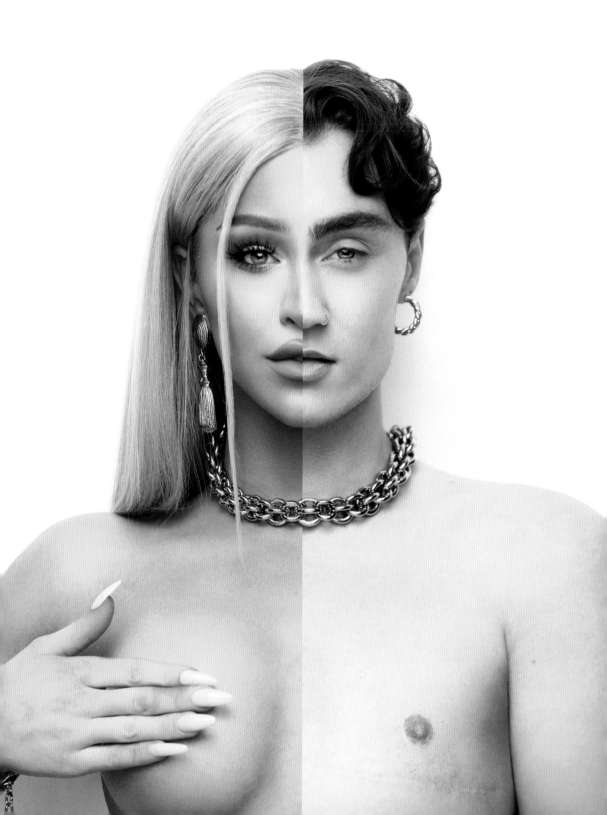

Visibility & Responsibility

When we think about what the transgender community needs most in order to make progress in this world, it's visibility. A lot of trans people are out and proud and loud, and a lot of them aren't. Who is responsible for making us more visible as a community, and what, exactly, does visibility entail?

GOTTMIK: If we're going to normalize the trans experience for the wider public, what we need is visibility and representation. We need more trans characters on TV shows and in movies and books. We need celebrities to be loud and proud. It's so important for trans people to see themselves reflected in popular culture. That's what starts conversations, and that's what normalizes trans people to the masses.

There's been progress in this area recently, but I think we need even more roles for queer characters and trans characters—that aren't sad. A lot of the time, the queer person's life is tragic, which is not helping our cause. We need characters who are living full and complex lives.

When a show with queer characters does come out, it's so helpful to watch it, support it, and post about it on social media if that's your thing. If the show does well, then whoever made it will be like, *Oh, showing the trans experience worked!* and they'll make other shows like it.

GIGI: Yes.

GOTTMIK: The straight, white cis male behind the desk in Hollywood is looking at the numbers. If nobody watches, they're going to remember that. So even if you hate the show and you think the characters are dumb, we should all be supporting any story about queer people.

GIGI: Yes.

GOTTMIK: Get obsessed, you know? Talk about it, post about it, comment on it, like it. That's not very hard to do. Just whip out your phone. There are times when I have not necessarily loved the show or the trans character, but I still go to the show's page and like it and comment on it. The cool thing is that you can see all the other comments of your fellow trans people when you do that. You can feel the community spirit and be happy about progress, even if the show isn't your thing. Everybody has preferences. Like with *Drag Race,* for example, I know that if somebody's not into me, they'll be into the next trans guy, and that's great.

GIGI: *Drag Race* took a chance on you.

GOTTMIK: Yes, they definitely took a risk putting me on the show. They didn't cast any openly trans guys until me. And the risk ended up working, only because the people who watched the show were so supportive and amazing. And now they're casting so many trans people and uplifting so many trans voices. Fans were so supportive of my journey on the show, and it was the best thing in the world, because I knew it meant that there would be more trans guys after me.

GIGI: One hundred percent. Since you were the first, did you feel a sense of responsibility to represent the community in a positive light?

GOTTMIK: I mean, I'm a perfectionist, so I definitely wanted to say the right things. But I realized that when I was just having fun and being myself was when everything was clicking and flowing and I was actually making connections that were allowing me to have conversations about things I care about, which is ultimately a lot more interesting than trying to stand on a soapbox and preach.

GIGI: You were so good. You'd never been on TV, and you were such a natural.

GOTTMIK: No, I had never been on TV. I was a makeup artist.

GIGI: But you were a fierce character behind the camera, too.

GOTTMIK: Oh yes. Even when I was doing makeup, I was loud and crazy and thriving off creative energy. I love that now I can do my art and wear it in front of the camera. It's so great.

GIGI: Do you think that all trans people should be out and proud? Like, is it everyone's responsibility to be visible?

GOTTMIK: If it's safe for them to do so, then yes.

GIGI: Right, your personal safety should come before everything else, of course.

GOTTMIK: If you don't have a strong support system around you, and if you live in a place that isn't accepting of the queer community, then I would say that being visible should not be your number one priority.

GIGI: Yes, one hundred percent.

GOTTMIK: For me, I love being visible. I mean, I was on a reality show, so of course I love it! But I don't necessarily feel that way all the time. It's an emotional roller coaster. Sometimes, I do think, *I wish I could go through the world and be perceived as a regular cis guy and just live my life.* But then, that might not even be completely true, because I'd miss the queer community, which is everything to me. And I love being able to tell my story, and I feel so lucky that I can reach a lot of people. Whenever I find out that I've helped someone on their journey by sharing my story, I feel honored to be out and proud.

GIGI: I think if you have any inkling that you might want to share your story publicly, then do it if you can, because it's very rewarding. You will hear from people; you will help people; you might save people's lives. You don't need to be on TV or on YouTube to share. Just posting about it on Facebook is huge.

GOTTMIK: Yes. Every voice counts.

GIGI: How visible you want to be is a personal choice. On the other side of the visibility spectrum from me, there's a girl I know named … we'll call her Sylvia. She started following me and then we got close online. She just had her gender confirmation surgery, and she is the most stealth, under-the-radar angel I know, and she's so happy that way. She'll go to gay bars. She's a part of the community, but she just does not want to scream it from the rooftops. She doesn't want to talk about trans issues. She doesn't want to be a trans voice. And I think that's fine. Not everyone is just able to handle the criticism or be out and proud and loud. Some people are just quiet people. Sylvia is one of those.

GOTTMIK: I totally get that, but I also think that if everyone did that, it would be bad. We'd all be invisible. Which would make it impossible to move forward. We want people to hear us and see us. We don't want to be hiding in the shadows.

GIGI: I totally hear you.

GOTTMIK: My hope for the future of the trans community is that we just dominate. I want us to become louder and prouder. I want more laws passed in our favor. We move forward; we move back; we move forward. That's the way of things. It swings like a pendulum. My hope is that we don't swing back too far. I want us to keep moving toward positivity and acceptance. At the end of the day, my hope is that we do everything we can to help the younger generations.

   In the media, I want to see more authentic trans characters. The word *authenticity* is cringe-worthy, but it's the right word. I want people watching to identify in a real way with the trans characters they see on TV. And I want trans people to feel like they can become anything they want, without limits. I want them all to feel less alone.

GIGI: If we have more representation in the media, then the people in this country who aren't exposed to trans people at all will begin to see it as normal.

GOTTMIK: And the less likely they are to be scared of a trans girl in the women's restroom. When people see girls like you getting married, Gigi, and being such a gorgeous example of kindness and pride, their minds start to change. They're like, "Oh, we're the same."

GIGI: It's amazing how much progress we've made in the last few decades.

GOTTMIK: Yes, and we're going to keep pushing forward. We're going to keep fighting. We're going to keep normalizing the trans experience. So, everyone's going to have to get into it or get lost.

Stay
Hopeful

with Sarah McBride

PHOTO BY **B PROUD**

For the transgender community, this is a moment of both pain and progress. More and more trans people are coming out at every age and in every community. Trans-inclusive policies have advanced in workplaces across the country and at the local, state, and federal level. Trans people are reaching new heights in business, in culture and the arts, and in politics—all of which seemed almost impossible just a decade ago.

At the same time, though, we are facing unprecedented challenges. Anti-trans laws are passing in states across the country, each one seeming to out-do the last in cruelty and in consequences. The epidemic of violence—particularly against Black transgender women—continues to grow. It seems like every time we turn on the television or open social media we're witnessing a new political attack or watching people devoid of experience debate our existence and our basic human rights.

It's exhausting, plain and simple.

As the first openly trans state senator in the country and the nation's highest-ranking out transgender elected official, I have a front row seat to all of it, the good and the bad. There's no question that being in this role creates unique pressures and responsibilities as both a trans person and as an elected

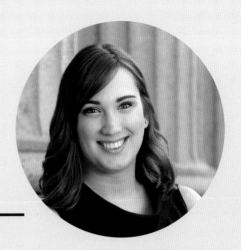

official. Ultimately, though, the mere fact that I have the opportunity to serve in public office demonstrates how lucky I am.

For those of us who are lucky enough to be living our truth and pursuing our dreams all at the same time, we must remember that we are only true trailblazers if we actually leave a trail behind us for others to follow. I'm not doing my job if I'm leaving a "me"-sized hole in the wall. It's critical that I help to bring down the wall.

As exhausting and frightening as this moment for trans people is, I remain hopeful. With those extra responsibilities that come with being a trans person in politics, come the

inspiring opportunities to meet people throughout our community. What I've seen is that our community is diverse, vibrant, and resilient. I've seen that we are organic agents of change, opening hearts and changing minds through our presence. Indeed, the change we seek will not come from politicians or public figures alone. It will come as more and more trans people open hearts and change minds in their neighborhoods, schools, workplaces, and faith communities. Having met so many members of our community, I am aware of how powerful we are, and this gives me immense hope for the future.

About the Authors

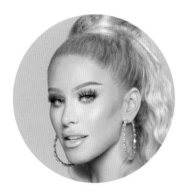

As a transgender woman, **Gigi Loren Lazzarato Getty** (better known as **Gigi Gorgeous**) inspires and entertains with her stories and larger-than-life personality. She's an actress, activist, author, and media personality who has appeared in *The New York Times, People, The Hollywood Reporter,* and more. She has graced the covers of *The Advocate* and *FASHION* magazine and has been named to the *Forbes 30 Under 30* and *Time's 25 Most Influential People on the Internet* lists. Her story was chronicled in the documentary *This Is Everything: Gigi Gorgeous,* and she is the author of *He Said, She Said.* On top of all her success, she's a glowing newlywed and shares three cats with her husband, Nats Getty.

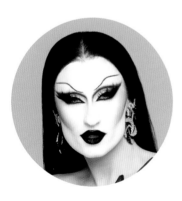

Gottmik (**Kade Gottlieb**) is a drag performer, makeup artist, author, and trans rights activist. The first openly trans man to compete on *RuPaul's Drag Race,* he has since appeared in *Vogue, OUT, Allure, InStyle,* and *Paper,* among other publications. He starred in Versace's 2022 Holiday campaign, appeared in Volume 3 of Rihanna's Savage X Fenty show, and is the co-host of *No Gorge,* a podcast and YouTube show, with fellow drag artist Violet Chachki. As a professional makeup artist, he has worked with Cindy Crawford, Paris Hilton, Lizzo, RuPaul, Kim Petras, Lil Nas X, and others. He studied his craft at The Los Angeles Institute of Design & Merchandising (FIDM) in Los Angeles, CA.

Acknowledgments

GIGI

I'd like to acknowledge all the love and support from the trans and queer communities over the years, which helped make writing this book possible. My admiration for the trailblazers before me is out of this world!

Thank you to my supporters, some of whom have been with me since day one when I was growing up in Toronto. You have my whole heart. I am so grateful for your camaraderie, which has allowed me to live authentically.

And thank you to my devoted father, for never giving up on me even in the most trying times. I wouldn't be the person I am today without your guidance.

GOTTMIK

First and foremost, I would like to acknowledge my amazing fans and supporters who have stood with me through everything. Sharing my trans experience as openly and honestly as I have is not always easy, and behind closed doors, I can sometimes fall into a mental hole and not want to climb out. You have shown so much respect for me and my journey, and this support inspires me to stand back up and keep fighting every time I fall.

I would also like to acknowledge RuPaul and the amazing team at World of Wonder for giving me a platform to share my art and my story with the world in ways I never could have dreamed of.

Finally, I would like to acknowledge my incredible family—both chosen and biological—for allowing me to always be myself and encouraging every wildly chaotic dream I think of. I would never be who I am or where I am without you.

Resources

National LGBTQIA+ Organizations

Many organizations are working on the national level to support LGBTQIA+ people across the United States and even worldwide. Check out these groups for more information on how they can help.

- The Trevor Project: *thetrevorproject.org*
- GLAAD: *glaad.org*
- Trans Wellness Center: *mytranswellness.org*
- It Gets Better Project: *itgetsbetter.org*
- National Center for Transgender Equality: *transequality.org*
- Transgender Legal Defense & Education Fund: *transgenderlegal.org*
- Trans Lifeline: *translifeline.org*
- PFLAG (Parents, Families, and Friends of Lesbians and Gays): *pflag.org/our-story*

Our Recommended Doctors

We've heard amazing things about these doctors, but please do the research you need to find the right doctor for you. Our hope is for this list to set you on the right path.

Bottom Surgery for Women:
- Dr. Christine McGinn, New Hope, PA: *drchristinemcginn.com/drmcginn/*
- Dr. Marci Bowers, Burlingame, CA: *marcibowers.com/*
- Dr. Toby Melter, Scottsdale, AZ: *themeltzerclinic.com/*
- Dr. Pierre Brassard, Montreal, Canada: *grsmontreal.com/en/surgeons/1-dr-pierre-brassard.html*
- Dr. Jess Ting, New York, NY: *profiles.mountsinai.org/jess-ting*

Bottom Surgery for Men:
- Dr. Dev Gurjala, San Francisco & Los Angeles, CA: *alignsurgical.com/about/dr-dev-gurjala/*
- Dr. Marci Bowers, Burlingame, CA: *marcibowers.com/*
- Crane Center for Transgender Surgery, Austin, TX & San Francisco, CA: *cranects.com*

Top surgeons
- Dr. Scott Mosser, Gender Confirmation Center: *genderconfirmation.com/team/dr-scott-mosser/*
- Dr. Daniel A. Medalie, Cleveland Plastic Surgery: *clevelandplasticsurgery.com/dr-medalie/*

FFS:
- Dr. Harrison Lee, Beverly Hills, CA, & New York, NY: *harrisonleeplasticsurgeon.com*

Breast Augmentation:
- Dr. Eugene Kim, Beverly Hills, CA: *ekimplasticsurgery.com*

Hair Transplants:
- Dr. Craig Ziering, Beverly Hills, CA: *zieringmedical.com*

Transition Assistance Organizations

Here are some organizations that could potentially help you pay for some of the elements of your transition. Some offer funding for gender-affirming procedures, some help you change your name, and some give away free trans gear. Check out each one to find out the specifics.

- Genderbands: *genderbands.org*
- The Jim Collins Foundation: *jimcollinsfoundation.org*
- The LOFT LGBTQ+ Community Center: *loftgaycenter.org*
- Point of Pride: *pointofpride.org*
- Trans United with Family and Friends (TUFF): *transunitedfund.org*
- We Are Family Foundation: *wearefamilyfoundation.org*

Crowdfunding Organizations

Another popular option to fund your transition is using one of these crowdfunding sites:

- DonationTo: *donationto.com*
- Fundly: *fundly.com*
- GoFundMe: *gofundme.com*
- GoGetFunding: *gogetfunding.com*

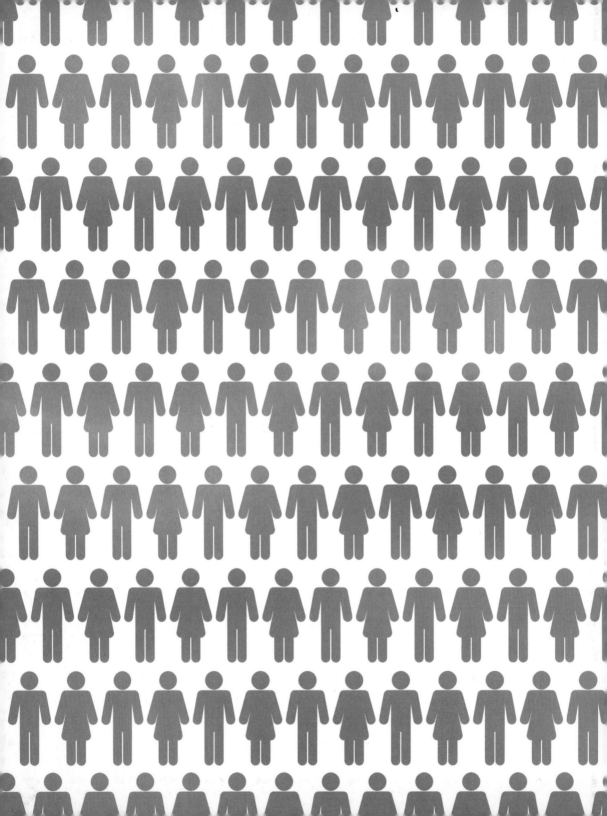